What Is Periodic Paralysis?

A Disease Like No Other

From

The Periodic Paralysis Network A.S.E.A. Series

Awareness ~ Support ~ Education ~ Advocacy

Volume Two

Susan Q. Knittle-Hunter

About the cover:
The silver background represents the color of potassium and the cream lettering represents paralysis awareness. These are the colors of our Periodic Paralysis awareness ribbon. The photo is of the author and was taken at a time when she was able to still propel herself in a wheelchair.

**What Is Periodic Paralysis?
A Disease Like No Other**
From
The Periodic Paralysis Network A.S.E.A. Series
Volume Two
By
Susan Q. Knittle-Hunter

Periodic Paralysis Network, Inc.
Sequim, Washington U.S.A.

All rights reserved. No part of the book may be reproduced or transmitted in any form or by any means, electronic or mechanical, including photocopying, recording or by any information storage or retrieval system, without written permission from the authors, except for the inclusion of brief quotations in a review.

Copyright © 2016
Library of Congress Cataloging-in-Publication Data:

**What Is Periodic Paralysis?
A Disease Like No Other**
From
The Periodic Paralysis Network A.S.E.A. Series
Volume Two
By
Susan Q. Knittle-Hunter

First Edition
Publish Date August 24, 2016

ISBN-13: 978-1536851731
ISBN-10: 1536851736

1. Andersen-Tawil Syndrome 2. Periodic Paralysis 3. Hypokalemia 4. Hyperkalemia 5. Normokalemia 6. Hypokalemic Periodic Paralysis 7. Hyperkalemic Periodic Paralysis
Printed in the United States of America.2016

Notice-Disclaimer
The ideas in this book are based on the authors' personal experiences with Periodic Paralysis, and as such are intended to provide only educational information on the covered subject to the reader. This book should not be used as a medical manual nor should this book be used as a diagnostic tool for Periodic Paralysis. The reader should consult a qualified health care professional or physician with expertise in Periodic Paralysis.

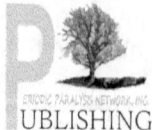

Periodic Paralysis Network, Inc. Publishing
Sequim, Washington U.S.A. 2016

This booklet is dedicated to my daughter Shari and to the members of our 'Periodic Paralysis Network Support, Education and Advocacy Group' for obvious reasons. May this booklet help you to be understood and believed by those in your life with whom you share it?

"Step into my shoes and walk the life I am living and if you get as far as I am, just maybe you will see how strong I really am."

~Unknown~

Table of Contents

About A.S.E.A.	vi
Preface	viii
Acknowledgements	ix
Introduction	13
What Is Periodic Paralysis?	17
What Are The Symptoms Of Periodic Paralysis?	29
What Are The Triggers Of Periodic Paralysis?	43
Relieving The Symptoms Of Periodic Paralysis	53
Handling The Episodes Of Periodic Paralysis	65
Diagnosing Periodic Paralysis	77
Complications Of Periodic Paralysis	91
Prognosis For Periodic Paralysis	121
Conclusion	129
Resources	140
About the Authors	141

About
The Periodic Paralysis Network
A.S.E.A. Series:

Awareness ~ Support ~ Education ~ Advocacy

Volume One

A Bill Of Rights For Periodic Paralysis Patients is the first volume in a series of booklets or handbooks being created, written and published by the Periodic Paralysis Network, Inc. (PPN). This series, called *The Periodic Paralysis Network A.S.E.A. Series*, is designed to bring awareness of Periodic Paralysis to the world; to provide support to individuals with all forms of Periodic Paralysis and their family members; to educate individuals about all aspects of Periodic Paralysis to include medical professionals and to provide advocacy for those with the condition and their family members and caregivers. The PPN was created and exists to provide **A**wareness, **S**upport, **E**ducation and **A**dvocacy to and for all individuals with Periodic Paralysis, their family members and caregivers as well as all medical professionals, thus the acronym A.S.E.A.

This second in the series is, *What Is Periodic Paralysis? A Disease Like No Other.*

Also By

Also by Susan Q. Knittle-Hunter & Calvin Hunter

Living With Periodic Paralysis: The Mystery Unraveled

*The Periodic Paralysis Guide And Workbook:
Be All You Can Be Naturally*

The A.S.E.A. series

A Bill Of Rights For Periodic Paralysis Patients

Also by Susan Q. Knittle-Hunter

Sotos Syndrome: A Tribute To Sandy

Also by Calvin Hunter

Moments In Time: At Home In The Woods

Preface

The Preface of a book gives the reader information about how the book came to be, where the idea originated. In the case of this booklet, my own family and the members of the 'Periodic Paralysis Network Support, Education and Advocacy Group' inspired, *What Is Periodic Paralysis? A Disease Like No Other*.

The members, now over 550 worldwide, share daily their heart-breaking and frustrating experiences. They relate frightening symptoms, years of painful and costly testing, a lack of being believed and abuse by doctors, denial of diagnoses and denial of proper treatment. These courageous and very ill people are under recognized; under diagnosed, misdiagnosed, misunderstood and mistreated by the medical professionals with whom they must deal and depend upon for their care. But to add insult to injury, this same treatment is also received from family members and friends who also tend to disbelieve the existence of the rare medical condition, Periodic Paralysis.

This booklet has been designed and written to share with family members, friends, teachers, coworkers and others who should know about and may want to know, the truth about this cruel disease.

For these reasons this booklet answering the question: "What is Periodic Paralysis?" has been created and written, by the PPN. The information used to describe and explain this disorder is referenced and can be found at the Periodic Paralysis Network, Inc. Website, Blog Articles, Discussion Groups and Books, to include: *Living With Periodic Paralysis: The Mystery Unraveled*, *The Periodic Paralysis Guide And Workbook: Be All You Can Be Naturally* and *A Bill Of Rights For Periodic Paralysis Patients*.

Acknowledgements

I would like to thank Calvin, my husband, for never doubting me, for believing me from the beginning, for supporting me and for saving my life. I would not be here today, writing our fourth book about Periodic Paralysis, if you had not desperately researched and discovered all of the natural ways to help me to manage the cruel and life-threatening symptoms including the paralytic episodes.

I also want to thank my daughter, Shari, for always being there for me. No matter how ill you may be, you always remember to call and check on me. Your attitude and strength are such an example to me and your love and support encourage me.

Rosie, without your friendship and inspiration, this book and the others, would not have been written. Thanks for believing in me and for being there for me.

Lastly, I would like to thank the members of our 'Periodic Paralysis Network Support, Education and Advocacy Group.' Each one of you has inspired me in more ways than you could possibly know. Thank you so much for your strength, words of encouragement, support and love. I could not do it all without each of you.

One

What Is Periodic Paralysis?
A Disease Like No Other

What Is Periodic Paralysis?

Imagine waking up one morning lying on your back, head slightly elevated, arms crossed and hands on your abdomen.
Imagine you attempt to open your eyes, but they will not open.
Imagine you try to move your arms and legs but they will not move.
Imagine you try to speak, but your mouth and tongue will not move.
Imagine your heart is beating fast, every few beats you feel palpitations.
Imagine you choke at times.
Imagine your chest muscles are very weak making it difficult to breathe.
Imagine you stop breathing, periodically.
Imagine you can hear everything going on around you.
Imagine staying that way for many hours and several times a day.
Imagine going to many doctors over many years and the tests come back normal and the doctors tell you it is all in your head.
Imagine taking twenty years or more to get a diagnosis, if you get one at all.
Imagine that your muscles get progressively and permanently weakened.
Imagine you can no longer work or take care of your family.
Imagine no one believes you, especially family, friends, doctors.
Imagine that nearly all medications cause these symptoms.
Imagine very few doctors know about this condition.
Imagine there are no cures and basically nothing doctors can do.
You have just entered the cruel world of Periodic Paralysis.
You are alone in the dark...
But there is hope...

Introduction

I would like to begin this book by introducing myself. I am Susan Q. Knittle-Hunter, the Co-Founder, Co-Creator and Managing Director of the Periodic Paralysis Network, Inc. I recently wrote the verse on the opposite page to bring awareness to Periodic Paralysis. The issues and concepts in the poem will be addressed in this booklet, which is designed to educate others about this little known and poorly understood disease.

I am diagnosed with a form of Periodic Paralysis called Andersen-Tawil Syndrome. It is the most rare and most serious form of the disease. I was sixty-two years old when I finally received my diagnosis after over 50 years of experiencing symptoms. I was misdiagnosed and mistreated with drugs I did not need, which made me worse as my health continued to decline. As new symptoms developed from the drugs, I received new diagnoses and more medications to treat the new symptoms. Eventually, I began to have full-body, paralytic episodes that involved my heart, breathing, blood pressure, oxygen levels, and much more. Trips to the hospital in the ambulance involved more drugs, near death experiences and no clear diagnosis.

On my own, after much research, I discovered I had Periodic Paralysis. I set out to get a diagnosis and eventually did, only to discover there was no cure and no way to stop my episodes of paralysis, which were now four or five times a day lasting for several hours at a time. I sought out any information I could find to know what to do. I found very little help, even from the groups who were supposed to be helping those of us with Periodic Paralysis. I saw many specialists as I continued to worsen, with no answers for controlling my disabling symptoms.

Finally, in desperation, Calvin, my husband, researched until he found some natural ways to help me. He changed my diet and helped me to discover the things that were causing my symptoms called triggers. After several months my episodes were greatly reduced. I was still very ill but felt a need to help others and share what we had learned so we decided to create our own website.

Over the past five years we have grown into a large forum with a website; a support, education and advocacy group with over 550 members worldwide, four more distinct discussion groups to include genealogy, genetics and caregivers; a learning center; a blog with over 130 articles and we have written three books about Periodic Paralysis (the only books written about it). This book is our fourth book and just as the other three, is written because there is a need to educate others and bring awareness of Periodic Paralysis to the world.

As discussed in the Preface and for the reasons listed, there was and is a great need for a booklet that can explain the important aspects of Periodic Paralysis in simple terms and how they relate personally to and for each individual with this disabling condition.

Some of the issues that are covered include but are not limited to, what Periodic Paralysis is and what it is not, how it is diagnosed, how it is treated, what the symptoms are, what causes the symptoms, what does an episode of paralysis look like, what is the prognosis and what kind of complications can occur. For each of these issues there is space for personal information to be included as needed to further explain how the disease affects each individual before the book is passed to a family member, neighbor, doctor or teacher. Each concept is described and explained based on the true and actual history, experiences and needs of individuals with Periodic Paralysis.

Periodic Paralysis is a multifaceted, complex, perplexing, complicated and overwhelming condition, which is very misunderstood by most doctors around the world, let alone patients with it and their friends and family members. The varying words, phrases and medical terms associated with it are difficult to pronounce and spell and even more difficult to understand. This book is an attempt to write about this very difficult and little understood disease in terms that are easy to understand and in an organized manner for better comprehension for those who need to or desire to know about it.

Hopefully, this information will bring about awareness of these issues and educate everyone who has the occasion to read this booklet. More information and referencing can be found at the Periodic Paralysis Network Inc Website, Blog Articles, discussion groups and books; *Living With Periodic Paralysis: The Mystery Unraveled* and *The Periodic Paralysis Guide And Workbook: Be The Best You Can Be Naturally* and *A Bill Of Rights For Periodic Paralysis Patients*. Links to these are at the back of the book.

What Is Periodic Paralysis?

Some Basic Facts

Periodic Paralysis is a little known and very misunderstood medical condition characterized by episodes of muscle weakness or paralysis, without the loss of sensation or feeling while still remaining conscious. While in an episode an individual can and does still hear everything happening around them and can feel everything that is done to them. It is very rare that one loses consciousness during an attack.

Periodic Paralysis can manifest in several forms and is a very misunderstood condition that is usually extremely difficult to diagnose. It can be progressive, debilitating, disabling and can even cause an early and unexpected death if not treated appropriately.

Many things can cause or trigger the symptoms including certain foods, exercise, stress, medications, temperature extremes, sleep and much more. The triggers cause potassium to shift in the body in abnormal ways, causing the symptoms, weakness and paralysis.

The Specific Facts

Periodic Paralysis Is A Medical Condition Like No Other

Periodic Paralysis (PP) is a very rare medical condition that is not like any other disorder. It is very unique; very different. It is not a neurological disease, nor an autoimmune disease, nor a disease of the mitochondria, nor an endocrine myopathy, nor is it a form of Muscular Dystrophy. It is in a category all of its own and needs to be treated in non-conventional ways. This means it must be treated differently than any other disease or illness.

PP Is A Medical Condition Known By Many Names

Periodic Paralysis (PP) is also known as Familial Periodic Paralysis and Myoplegia Paroxysmalis Familiaris. There are several forms of PP and each has its own name. These will be discussed later.

PP Is A Medical Condition That Is Inherited

Periodic Paralysis is an extremely rare condition that one has at birth. A person is born with PP. It is passed from either the mother or the father or from both parents to any of the children, male or female.

PP Is A Medical Condition Caused By A Mutation In A Gene

Periodic Paralysis is caused by a permanent flaw, alteration or mistake in the sequence of the DNA of a gene. Each person is born with about 20,000 genes, which are divided among 23 chromosomes. Slight differences in the genes are what make us distinct from one another. Larger differences or defects in the genes can create medical illnesses, diseases or conditions. This is what causes Periodic Paralysis in most individuals.

PP Is An Ion Channelopathy

An alteration in certain genes can cause what is known as an ion channelopathy. Periodic Paralysis was one of the first ion channelopathies recognized in 1971. An ion channelopathy is a dysfunction of an ion channel, a microscopic tunnel in the cells of muscles called muscle fibers. Particles of potassium, sodium, chloride and calcium, which are electrically charged, known as ions, flow in and out of the cells. They regulate the contraction or tightening and relaxation of the muscle. A problem with the flow can cause paralysis and other symptoms.

PP Is A Mineral Metabolic Disorder

Metabolism is related to all of the chemical reactions in the human body that keeps it stabilized and balanced. A metabolic disorder is an imbalance of the chemicals. Ions, also know as minerals and electrolytes, are related to and part of the chemical processing that occurs in the body. A mineral metabolic disorder is abnormal levels of the ions, minerals and electrolytes. Periodic Paralysis is an imbalance of potassium and the other electrolytes, therefore Periodic Paralysis, which is a channelopathy, is also considered to be mineral metabolic disorder.

PP Is A Medical Condition Related To Faulty Potassium Flow

Potassium is the basic mineral responsible for the symptoms and periods of paralysis involved in Periodic Paralysis. Potassium flows improperly in or out of the ion channels or fibers of the muscle cells. Depending on the form of PP, the muscles will tighten or loosen causing muscle weakness or paralysis.

PP Is A Medical Condition With Symptoms That Begin In The Cells

So, Periodic Paralysis is a condition in which the symptoms of intermittent periods of paralysis, or muscle weakness, begin within the muscle cells of the body.

PP Is A Medical Condition With Many Forms

The most common forms or types of Periodic Paralysis are listed below along with the description of how the paralysis and other symptoms result.

Hypokalemic Periodic Paralysis (HypoPP or HypoKPP)

Also known as Westphall Disease, in HypoKPP, paralysis results from potassium moving from the blood into muscle cells in an abnormal way due to the calcium channel not signaling for appropriate release of calcium. It is associated with low levels of potassium in the blood (hypokalemia) during paralytic episodes.

Hyperkalemic Periodic Paralysis (HyperPP or HyperKPP)

In HyperKPP, also known as Gamstorp Disease, Paralysis results from sodium flowing into the cells because the channel remains open inappropriately. It is associated with high levels of potassium in the blood (hyperkalemia) during paralytic episodes.

Andersen-Tawil Syndrome (ATS)

With ATS, also known as Long QT Syndrome 7, paralysis results when the channel does not open properly; potassium cannot leave the cell. This disrupts the flow of potassium ions in skeletal and cardiac muscle. During paralytic episodes, ATS can be associated with low potassium, high potassium or shifts within the normal (normokalemia) ranges of potassium. An arrhythmia, long Qt interval heartbeat, is associated with ATS as well as certain characteristics, such as webbed or partially webbed toes, crooked little fingers and dental anomalies.

Normokalemic Periodic Paralysis (NormoPP or NormoKPP)

Paralysis results when potassium shifts within in normal ranges. This can happen in any form of Periodic Paralysis; Hypokalemic Periodic Paralysis, Hyperkalemic Periodic Paralysis, Normokalemic Periodic Paralysis and Andersen-Tawil Syndrome. The paralysis may result from the shifting itself, rather than low or high potassium or it may occur due to the shifting of the potassium, which can happen very quickly and is undetectable in lab testing.

Paramyotonia Congenita (PMC)

With PMC, also known as Von Eulenberg's Disease, the skeletal muscles can become stiff, tight, tense or contracted and weak when the sodium channels close much too slowly and the sodium, potassium, chloride and water continue to flow into the muscles. It is actually considered to be a form of Hyperkalemic Periodic Paralysis, however, the symptoms can appear from shifting of potassium into low or high ranges or even if potassium shifts within normal levels.

Thyrotoxic Periodic Paralysis (TPP)

In TPP, also known as Thyrotoxic Hypokalemic Periodic Paralysis, intermittent paralysis results from low potassium due to an overactive thyroid or hyperthyroidism. It can occur spontaneously or can result from a genetic mutation. Unlike the other forms of Periodic Paralysis, TPP can be treated and cured by removing or treating the thyroid.

Electrolyte Periodic Paralysis (EPP)

At the time this book is being written a new form of Periodic Paralysis is coming to light. It may be that any of the minerals or electrolytes may be shifting in error creating the symptoms and paralysis. Not much is know about it at this time.

The form of Periodic Paralysis I have is:
(You may add your personal information to share with others for their better understanding before you pass along this book.)

The General Facts

PP Is A Chronic Illness

This means:

The Symptoms of Periodic Paralysis last more than three months.

The symptoms of Periodic Paralysis last a lifetime.

Vaccines will not prevent Periodic Paralysis.

However, vaccines can harm those with Periodic Paralysis.

Medications will not cure Periodic Paralysis.

But, drugs and medications may harm those with it.

Periodic Paralysis will not disappear or go away no matter what we do!!!

PP Is An Invisible Illness

This means

'You look fine'

Periodic Paralysis shows no visible outward sign of the illness. Individuals look 'good' except for the intermittent episodes of paralysis or muscle weakness.

BUT

Periodic Paralysis is a chronic illness.

It lasts a lifetime, vaccines will not prevent it and drugs will not cure it.

AND

Periodic Paralysis significantly impairs and affects activities of normal daily living and most of those with it are considered disabled due to organ damage.

(One may end up using a cane, crutches or wheelchairs and may not be able to work due to progressive permanent muscle weakness, but they will still look 'normal.' Thus leaving others to wonder why they are using a cane or a wheelchair.)

Two

The Symptoms Of Periodic Paralysis

Periodic Paralysis Is More Than Just Periods Of Paralysis

The most obvious characteristic for each form of Periodic Paralysis is the episode of intermittent paralysis, but there are various ways in which the paralytic episodes can manifest themselves. Depending on the type of Periodic Paralysis and the potassium levels, which may be high, low or in normal ranges found in the blood serum and the speed with which the potassium shifts, the episodes or attacks can be markedly different.

Episodes may be as simple as dizziness, numbness or tingling, passing out, sudden dropping or falling to the ground or partial paralysis. This may include paralysis of just the legs, or maybe an arm or one side of the body. The episodes may be only muscle weakness, either full body or just a part of the body. They may be as serious as full body paralysis including dangerous heart arrhythmia, heart rate fluctuation, blood pressure fluctuations, choking, breathing difficulties, including the cessation of breathing and cardiac arrest and/or respiratory arrest, which can lead to death in some instances. Attacks may happen as often as several during a day or only one or two in a lifetime. They may happen suddenly or they may give a few warnings and happen gradually. They may change over time getting progressively worse or they may become less severe. It may happen that each episode is different or unique. They may last from just a few minutes to many hours or even last for days or weeks at a time. Some individuals with known genetic markers for Periodic Paralysis may never go into paralysis. Some may only experience a gradual and permanent muscle weakness. Regardless, an individual with Periodic Paralysis is usually a very unwell person because although the symptoms will come and go, the episodes usually do damage to the organs in the body, creating permanent disability and debilitation in many ways.

The following are just some of the symptoms characteristics and side effects that are related to and experienced with this rare medical condition. They may be seen before during or after an episode. They may also be seen or experienced at any time or are the result of the repeated episodes or just the nature of being a mineral metabolic disorder.

fast heartbeat - irregular heartbeat - slow heartbeat - high blood pressure - low blood pressure - pain - muscle weakness - fatigue - low oxygen - progressive permanent muscle weakness - breathing difficulties - choking - numbness - tingling - muscle cramping - muscle aches - muscle spasms - inability to open eyes - long QT heartbeat - slurring of words - headaches - inability to speak - vision issues - excessive thirst - increased urination - nausea - stomach cramps - blockage of intestines - chest pain - shortness of breath - irritability - anxiousness - sleepiness - confusion - lack of clear thinking - seizures - high potassium levels - low potassium levels - normal potassium levels - metabolic acidosis - partial paralysis - full-body paralysis - abortive attacks - disability - life-changing - co-existing conditions - possible death - exercise intolerance - inability to use anesthesia - odd side effects of drugs - opposite effects of drugs

An individual with Periodic Paralysis may experience most of these symptoms or only a few of them, depending on the form they have and the trigger or triggers.

The Symptoms Of Periodic Paralysis

Hypokalemic Periodic Paralysis

For those with Hypokalemic Periodic Paralysis (low potassium), which makes up about 70% of all cases, these are the symptoms normally seen.

Muscles: Fatigue, pain in the joints, muscle weakness, muscle weakness after exercise, muscle stiffness, muscle aches, muscle cramps, muscle contractions, muscle spasms, muscle tenderness, pins and needles sensation, eyelid myotonia (cannot open eyelid after opening and then closing them).

Digestion: Upset stomach, loss of appetite, vomiting, constipation, diarrhea, bloating of the stomach and full feeling in the stomach, blockage in the intestines called paralytic ileus.

Heart: Anxiousness, irregular and rapid heartbeat, angina, prominent U waves, inverted or flattened T waves, ST depression, elongated PR interval.

Kidneys: Severe thirst, increased urination, difficulty breathing, too slow or shallow breathing, lack of oxygen in the blood, sweating, increased blood pressure, metabolic acidosis.

Liver: The brain function becomes affected if the liver is involved causing irritability, decrease in concentration, lack of clear thinking, confusion, slurring of speech, seizures.

Paralysis: Episodic muscle weakness, episodic partial paralysis, episodic total paralysis, episodic flaccid paralysis (limp muscles, without tone).

Hyperkalemic Periodic Paralysis

For those with Hyperkalemic Periodic Paralysis (high potassium), which makes up about 15% of all cases, these are the symptoms normally seen.

Muscles: Fatigue, weakness, pins and needles, tingling or numbness in the extremities, muscle contraction, muscle rigidity, muscle cramps, muscles stiffness, muscle twitching, muscle cramping, reduced reflexes, muscle contraction involving tongue, tightness in legs, strange feeling in legs.

Digestion: Discomfort, nausea, vomiting, stomach cramps, diarrhea, vomiting.

Heart: Palpitations, chest pain, irregular heartbeat, slow heartbeat, weak pulse, absent pulse, heart stoppage, small P waves, tall T waves, QRS abnormality, P wave abnormality, QT lengthening, fast heartbeat.

Kidneys: Breathing problems, wheezing, shortness of breath, fast breathing, feeling hot, low blood pressure.

Liver: The brain function becomes affected: irritability, sleepiness, confusion, seizures, and loss of consciousness.

Paralysis: Episodic muscle weakness, episodic partial paralysis, episodic total paralysis.

Andersen-Tawil Syndrome

For those with Andersen-Tawil Syndrome, it is the most rare and the most serious form and accounts for about 10% of all cases of Periodic Paralysis. Potassium shifts in high and low ranges and also within normal ranges causing symptoms and paralysis. The symptoms normally seen are listed in the above two sections.

Two more components characterize ATS. They are distinctive crania-facial (head and face) and skeletal characteristics and long QT interval heartbeat with a predisposition toward life-threatening ventricular arrhythmia. However, affected individuals may express only one or two of the three components and they may be very subtle. Other characteristics and abnormalities are also associated with Andersen-Tawil Syndrome.

These physical abnormalities and characteristics associated with Andersen-Tawil Syndrome are as follows:

Characteristics and Features:

(May be very subtle, partial or seen in 'unaffected' family members)

Skeletal: Delayed bone age (slowed degree of maturation of child's bones), short stature, scoliosis (curved spine).

Dental: Hypodontia (born with missing teeth), persistent primary dentition (adults still have some baby teeth).

Hands and Feet: Brachydactyly (unusually short fingers), brachydactyly type D (clubbed thumbs) (characterized by a slightly shorter thumb that is round in section and larger at the end), clinodactyly (inward curvature/ 5th fingers), syndactyly (webbing between fingers or between 2nd and 3rd toes).

Face: Short palpebral fissures (short opening for the eyes between the eyelids), ocular hypertelorism (widely spaced eyes), microcephaly (abnormal smallness of the head), broad nasal root (wide space between the inner corners of eyes), broad forehead (increased distance between the two sides of the forehead or top to bottom of forehead), malar hypolasia (small cheek bones), micrognathia (short jaw), prognathism (protruding jaw), ptosis (an abnormally low position (drooping) of the upper eyelid), low set ears.

Mouth: Small mandible (lower jaw in which the lower teeth reside and chin), hypoplasia of maxilla (small upper jaw), cleft palate (born with a fissure in the roof of the mouth), high arched palate (roof of the mouth is high).

Joints: Joint laxity (looseness of the muscles and soft tissue surrounding a joint).

Heart: Ventricular arrhythmia, abnormal heart rhythm, long QT syndrome (increased time needed for heart to recharge after each heartbeat), irregular heartbeat, fainting caused by irregular heartbeat.

Executive Functioning Disorder (EF) can accompany ATS. There are three primary layers of executive functions: Self-regulation, organization and high order reasoning skills. It is associated with many disabilities: Attention Deficit Hyperactivity Disorder, Learning Disabilities, Tourette Syndrome, Obsessive Compulsive Disorder, autism, depression.

Normokalemic Periodic Paralysis

Normokalemic Periodic Paralysis is a form of Periodic Paralysis in which the potassium does not shift out of normal ranges, however an individual becomes partially or fully paralysed intermittently. The paralysis results from the actual shifting of the potassium. This may happen in any form of Periodic Paralysis and there are also specific genetic mutations responsible for this. The symptoms normally seen are a combination of the same myriad of symptoms seen in either Hypokalemic Periodic Paralysis or Hyperkalemic Periodic Paralysis.

Paramyotonia Congenita

One who suffers with Paramyotonia Congenita may experience a variety of symptoms, but usually the skeletal muscles can become stiff, tight, and tense or they can become contracted and weak. Due to the fact that PMC is actually considered to be a form of Hyperkalemic Periodic Paralysis, the symptoms will be the same as seen in Hyperkalemic Periodic Paralysis.

Thyrotoxic Periodic Paralysis

An individual with Thyrotoxic Periodic Paralysis typically suffers with symptoms exactly like

Hypokalemic Periodic Paralysis. They also have high levels of the thyroid hormone.

Abortive Attacks

Abortive attacks are periods of extended time anywhere from hours, days, weeks or months in which some individuals are totally debilitated by extreme muscle weakness without going into full paralysis. The previously described common symptoms may begin but the full attack or total paralysis may not occur. The person is left with severe weakness and other symptoms such as extreme fatigue. It is difficult to do anything physically and it also can affect cognition abilities, such as memory, thought processing and speech and some become very fragile emotionally. The individual may want to sleep and may have no appetite. In most cases the abortive attacks are totally debilitating and actually worse than the episodes of paralysis.

Description Of A Full-Body Episode

The following is a description of what it is like to be in a full-body, total, paralytic episode, involving the heart, breathing, choking and blood pressure. The author wrote this passage before she knew about Periodic Paralysis and did not understood what was happening to her. These episodes lasted for many hours at that time. Fears of the unknown and possible death are large components of a paralytic episode.

Alone in the Dark

"It is early morning when I awaken. I am lying on my back with my head slightly elevated on my pillow with my arms crossed and my hands on my abdomen. I attempt to open my eyes, but they will not open. I try to move my arms and legs but they will not move. I try to speak, but my mouth is open and will not move. My tongue is thick and dry and will not move. I am breathing very shallow breaths in and out of my mouth. My heart is beating very quickly and every few beats I feel palpitations. Occasionally, my throat attempts to swallow but cannot and I choke making a gurgling sound as my head thrusts back against my pillow.

Oh no. It is happening again. I am afraid. What is this? What is happening to me? Will I stay this way this time? Will my heart slow down? Will the palpitations get worse? Will I choke to death? My breathing has stopped. I cannot take a breath. Am I dying? Someone please help me get through this. A few seconds go by and finally I feel a little air enter my lungs; a shallow breath, then another. Thank goodness. Does Calvin know this is happening again? I cannot tell him. I am unable to wake him up because I am not able to speak, nor can I move. But, I need him to listen to my heart, to watch my breathing and to make sure I do not choke. I am so afraid.

What time is it? How long have I been like this? How long will it last this time? I have an itch on my face but am unable to scratch it. Oh no, my breathing stops again. A few more seconds go by, finally another shallow breath. My eyes begin to sting and I feel tears run down my face toward my ears.

I am so alone. I have never felt so alone; been so alone. Please, please make this stop.

Why is this happening to me? Should I go to the hospital? After all, I am paralyzed. I thought doctors take care of people who are paralyzed. I wish Calvin would wake up and call an ambulance, but at the same time I am afraid to go to the ER. They treated me so bad the last 3 times I went. They treated me like I was faking these episodes. Why would I do that? Once they told me that I was having seizures. Another time it was possibly my heart. The last time they gave me a medication that almost killed me. I immediately went unconscious. Calvin had to remove me before I was discharged before they could do it again. What would happen if I went again to the hospital like this? I am afraid to go to but I want help. I need help. There has to be someone who can help me...

My eyelids are still closed. I am unable to move yet. My heart still races and my breathing remains shallow. I am lucky to be able to hear. Calvin is softly breathing as he sleeps next to me. The heater clicks on. A bird is singing outside the window. Our cat scratches in his litter box. Life is continuing around me.

I am alone in the dark. (June 2010)"

~Susan Q. Knittle-Hunter~

My symptoms, episodes and characteristics include:

(You may add your personal information to share with others for their better understanding before you pass along this book.)

The Symptoms Of Periodic Paralysis

Three

The Triggers Of Periodic Paralysis

Many Things Can Cause The Symptoms Of Periodic Paralysis

The episodes of paralysis or muscle weakness and other symptoms are created, triggered or set off by many things, including food and drugs. The following is a comprehensive list. These are not 'set in stone' and can cross over among the different forms of Periodic Paralysis. As a rule, anything that causes adrenaline to rise in the body can set an episode into motion.

The Common Triggers Of Hypokalemic Periodic Paralysis

The triggers usually responsible for causing potassium to shift in Hypokalemic Periodic Paralysis are:

Eating a large amount of carbohydrates in a meal
Eating a meal with too much salt
Stress (good or bad)
Vigorous exercise
Resting after exercise
After lengthy periods of inactivity (traveling in a car)
Cold
Infections
Epinephrine/adrenaline
Insulin
Pregnancy
Surgery
Anesthesia
Glucose (Dextrose) IV
Saline (Sodium) IV
Steroids

The Common Triggers Of Hyperkalemic Periodic Paralysis

The triggers usually responsible for causing potassium to shift in Hyperkalemic Periodic Paralysis are:

Ingesting too much potassium in food, supplements or medications
Stress (good or bad)
Rest after exercise
Fatigue
Fasting
Possibly low blood sugar
Alcohol
Pregnancy
Contaminated air such as smoking
Weather changes
Cholinesterase inhibitors
Depolarizing muscle relaxants

The Common Triggers Of Paramyotonia Congenita

The triggers usually responsible for causing potassium to shift in Paramyotonia Congenita are:

Exercise
Exertion
Repetitious movement
Cold
Sleeping in
Possibly all triggers for Hyperkalemic Periodic Paralysis

Other Triggers For Periodic Paralysis Can Include:

Diet: Diet can be one of the biggest contributors to episodes of paralysis.

Simple carbohydrates: sugar, white flour and more
Complex carbohydrates: some grains, wheat, rye and more
Meat: mostly red meats
Salt
Caffeine
MSG
Alcohol
Large meals
Gluten
Processed foods
Food dyes
Food additives
Food preservatives
Meat or dairy products with hormones, and antibiotics
Fruits and vegetables with pesticides
Drinking water with hormones, antibiotics, pesticides or traces of any drugs (most drinking water, even bottled water)

Sleep: All aspects of sleep may set episodes into motion:

Falling asleep
During sleep
Waking up

Other:
Dehydration
Fasting

Sitting too long
Changes in the weather
Fatigue
Heat
Cold
Electromagnetic Force (EMF's)
Menstrual cycle
Pregnancy
Surgery
Infections, viruses
Immunizations, vaccinations
Sudden or strobing lights, sounds, movements (touch, sound or vision)
Chemicals (sensitivity)

Exercise: Some individuals have no problem with exercise but others may not be able to tolerate any type of exercise or very little exercise. This is called 'exercise intolerance.' Episodes may develop soon after or the next day.

Rest after exercise: May set an episode into motion.

Unknown: One can follow all the rules and still have episodes for unknown reasons.

Over-the-counter medications: Most over the counter medications, can set muscle weakness or paralysis into motion for people with Periodic Paralysis. The following is a list of some known offenders.

Eye drops
Glycerin enemas
NSAID's
Cough syrups

Compounds or Chemicals: Products with the following ingredients should be avoided:

Sodium Hydroxide
Edetate Disodium
Stearic Acid

They may be in any of the following: Lotions, oils, hair dyes or colors, antiperspirants, enemas, suppositories, soaps, shampoos, shaving creams, foams, toothpastes, deodorants, beauty products, skincare products, cosmetic products, bath salts, emollients, ointments, creams, hair sprays, perfumes, colognes, powders, hair gels, oils, tonics, mousse.

Drugs: Many, many drugs can set muscle weakness or paralysis into motion for people with Periodic Paralysis. There are also other serious reasons for those with this condition to avoid most drugs, medications or pharmaceuticals.

The two most common issues with drugs or pharmaceuticals for individuals with Periodic Paralysis are a paradoxical reaction and an idiosyncratic reaction. These are both serious effects. If one has a paradoxical reaction to a medication it means that the opposite of what is supposed to happen will occur. A pill to stop pain may actually cause pain, for instance. If someone develops an idiosyncratic reaction, side effects may occur which have never happened previously to anyone who has taken the drug. The effects will be very extreme and unusual. They could be harmful or even cause death. This will be discussed in more depth later in the book.

If one must take a drug, it is better to begin with ¼ of a normal dose to make sure it will be tolerated.

Saline drips, glucose infusion: If an IV is needed, mannitol can be used (or diluted solutions in extreme cases) (excluding HyperKPP)
Oral or Intravenous Corticosteroids
Muscle relaxers
Beta blockers
Tranquilizers
Pain killers (analgesics)
Antihistamines (except HyperKPP)
Puffers for asthma
Antibiotics
Cough syrups
Eye drops to dilate eyes
Contrast dye for MRI's
Lidocaine
Anesthetics
Epinephrine (Can sometimes help symptoms of Hyperkalemic Periodic Paralysis)
Adrenaline (Can sometimes help symptoms of Hyperkalemic Periodic Paralysis)

For more information about the medications or drugs, which can cause muscle weakness, muscle paralysis, long QT interval hearts beats (ATS) and torsades de pointes (ATS) please go to:

http://www.periodicparalysisnetwork.com/pdf/What are the Periodic Paralysis Triggers.pdf

The Triggers Of Periodic Paralysis

My triggers include:
(You may add your personal information to share with others for their better understanding before you pass along this book.)

Four

Relieving The Symptoms Of Periodic Paralysis

There Is No Known Cure For Periodic Paralysis...

BUT, there are ways to manage or relieve some of the symptoms and reduce the number and severity of the episodes.

Once an individual is born with Periodic Paralysis he or she will have it their entire life. It will not go away, it will not be recovered from, remedied or cured. The genetic mutation will always be in the genes. No 'thinking good thoughts' or 'more exercise' or 'eating of bananas' or 'prayers' or 'good wishes' or 'meditation' or 'wearing of crystals' or 'trying harder' will make it go away. There is no 'quick fix,' 'magical cure,' 'healing medication,' or 'perfect treatment.' No one grows out of it.

However, there are things that can be done to treat or help to manage the symptoms and paralysis. There is HOPE that an individual can improve the quality of his or her life by reducing the symptoms and the number of paralytic episodes and the severity of them and therefore slowing the damage to the organs and gradual permanent muscle weakness. This can be done without drugs of any kind for most individuals.

This chapter contains the most important components for the relief, treatment or management of symptoms. It is based on and uses mostly natural methods and substances in order to reduce the attacks of paralysis and other symptoms. It is a great deal of work and a constant battle, however.

There are two parts or components to treating Periodic Paralysis. The first is doing what is necessary to avoid the symptoms and periods of paralysis and the second part is handling the symptoms and paralytic episodes once they begin. For the most part these can and should be done as naturally as possible.

Reducing Or Preventing The Symptoms

There are no two people with Periodic Paralysis who are exactly alike. Even members of the same family have triggers and symptoms that differ from each other, and their episodes are most likely different also. Each person must discover the things that work best for him or her. This takes a great deal of work and must be done by trial and error. Good record keeping is important.

The following is an outline of the best methods or plan used to reduce, avoid or prevent the symptoms and paralysis. Each paralytic episode causes more muscle and organ damage so it is necessary to do everything possible to stop the episodes.

Avoid All Known Triggers

The most obvious and common sense step that can easily be done to relieve our symptoms is to avoid the triggers known to cause them. Some are very obvious and others may take some time to discover. Sometimes a person may never know what sets an attack into motion. The previous chapter discussed the most obvious and common triggers.

Eat A pH Balanced Diet

Because Periodic Paralysis is a mineral metabolic disorder, individuals are prone to chronic metabolic acidosis. This is too much acidity in the body. Being too acidic can set symptoms and paralysis into motion. A pH balance of 70% alkaline and 30% acidity works the best. Some may also have the opposite, metabolic alkalinity, which is too much alkaline, so a pH balance diet can help with either issue.

Total Balance In Diet

'Balance' is the most important word in the diet plan. If just one thing is out of balance, it can mean the difference between life and death in some cases. Besides the 70/30 balances in our diet, the other elements in our body must be in balance also, especially the elements or minerals (sometimes called electrolytes). This is due to the fact that Periodic Paralysis is a mineral metabolic disorder and when the minerals are out of balance, paralysis will occur. Some of these elements are calcium, magnesium, sodium, potassium, chloride, and bicarbonate.

That being said, however, salt (sodium) may be a trigger for paralytic episodes for most individuals. Due to that fact many of us avoid it like the plague. If we do not eat any salt then our body will get out of balance and episodes of paralysis or other symptoms may develop. So we must carefully ingest some sodium for that balance.

This also includes natural sugar and some fats and oils. These are also needed in our body, but care must be given to how much we eat of them in our diet and which types. Natural sugars in fruits would be a better choice than white processed table sugar. Olive oil is a better choice than vegetable oil. Monounsaturated fats and polyunsaturated fats are a better choice than saturated fats.

Avoid Processed Foods

Processed foods contain high acidity, fillers, additives, dyes, sodium, sugar, gluten and more that are known triggers for most individuals who have Periodic Paralysis. Therefore they should be avoided.

Use Organic Foods

Organic foods are natural foods containing no pesticides, antibiotics, hormones or other harmful components. As already stated, these are triggers for most people with Periodic Paralysis. Non-organically grown vegetables and fruits will almost always contain pesticides. Non-organically raised animals pose some real problems. The dairy products and meat from these animals will contain a certain amount of antibiotics and hormones. If antibiotics or hormones are triggers for an individual, he or she may not be aware that those will be found in the milk, cheese or meat they eat. Without realizing it they may be ingesting them, thus creating episodes of paralysis and not knowing why.

Drink Distilled Water

Most water, even bottled water, contains pesticides, antibiotics, hormones, opiates, anti-depressants and other drugs which are impossible to filter out as well as jet fuel and other harmful contaminants. These can all create the shifting of potassium or other symptoms. The distilling process removes these things from the water. The trace minerals that are also distilled out may need to be obtained in foods or with natural supplements.

Use Organic Natural Supplements

Most supplements contain fillers, additives, dyes and more. It is important to purchase and use only natural, organic supplements, as explained previously, to avoid the possibility of developing symptoms and paralysis.

Stay Well Rested

It is extremely important for individuals with Periodic Paralysis to stay well rested. Otherwise an individual's body becomes stressed and stress equals paralysis. A full night of sleep is essential. Unfortunately, many are affected by paralysis at night because different phases of sleep are a trigger. Falling asleep, during sleep and waking up may trigger a paralytic episode. It is best to do everything possible to make those times, stress free, comfortable and temperature controlled to make it less likely to trigger an episode.

Stay Well Hydrated

Being chronically ill leaves individuals more susceptible to dehydration, which is when the body loses more liquid than it takes in. Less water and fluids affects the balance of the electrolytes and prevents the organs from working properly. This creates an imbalance, which creates stress in the body. As we know, stress can trigger paralysis.

The most important way to stay hydrated is to drink plenty of water and other healthy liquids. Sports drinks or fruit juices contain a great deal of sugar and need to be avoided. Vegetable juices contain a great deal of sodium or if they are low sodium use added potassium for better flavor so should be used with care.

Avoid Physical Exercise And Exertion

Most individuals with all forms of Periodic Paralysis usually avoid physical exercise, physical exertion, weight lifting, heavy labor and physical therapy. This is due to exercise intolerance and/or gradual permanent muscle weakness (PMW). The recurring episodes of paralysis cause damage to the muscles, thus creating exercise intolerance leading to gradual muscle weakness and over time permanent muscle weakness (PMW) results. The damage done to the muscles is written about much less often than the episodes of partial or full paralysis in articles or studies about Periodic Paralysis. The information available, however, indicates that PMW is seen in all forms of Periodic Paralysis; Hypokalemic Periodic Paralysis, Hyperkalemic Periodic Paralysis, Normokalemic Periodic Paralysis or Andersen-Tawil Syndrome. Progressive muscle damage is also seen in all forms and it is irreparable. It cannot be reversed.

Avoid Heat And Cold

Maintaining a balanced temperature in the environment is important for people with Periodic Paralysis. If an individual gets overheated or chilled, the body becomes stressed and can trigger a paralytic episode. Being prepared for transitional times is the best idea.

Avoid Stress

Stress, whether good stress or bad stress, is a serious issue for individuals with Periodic Paralysis. Potassium drops when the body is stressed. The shift creates symptoms and paralysis in all forms and needs to be avoided.

Monitor All Vitals

The vital signs, including blood pressure, heart rate, body temperature, oxygen levels, glucose levels, potassium levels, pH levels, and more should be monitored closely every day and throughout each day and when symptoms begin. Some of the tools necessary to do this include the potassium reader, finger pulse oximeter, blood sugar monitor, wrist blood pressure monitor, stethoscope, thermometer and a digital pH balance reader or litmus paper. Changes and imbalances detected indicate potassium and electrolyte shifts. In this way some episodes can be stopped or treated before they become too serious and aide in knowing what method to use or when and if an individual may need emergency care.

Potassium: To Take Or Not To Take?

Most people with Hypokalemic Periodic Paralysis use potassium supplementation in some manner. Due to the fact that Periodic Paralysis symptoms and episodes of paralysis occur due to abnormal levels and shifting of potassium, there is a misconception that everyone needs to take potassium in some form daily. This is not the case. Unless it is known that an individual's potassium level is actually low (at any given moment), a person may not need potassium supplementation. Those with Hyperkalemic Periodic Paralysis must avoid potassium. If potassium does not shift out of normal levels as in Normokalemic Periodic Paralysis or Andersen-Tawil Syndrome, potassium is not needed.

Potassium comes in many forms so those who do need to take it must know which form and compound is the best for their particular symptoms.

Carbonic Anhydrase Inhibitor: Use Or Not?

There is much controversy in the Periodic Paralysis community and among doctors about the use of carbonic anhydrase inhibitors. There are three forms of the same drug that are prescribed, which are diuretics and each is sulfa-based. They are touted to help all forms of Periodic Paralysis, but each form has a different way in which the movement of potassium causes the symptoms, so it is nearly impossible that one type of drug could treat the symptoms for all forms.

Only some mutations are helped with the drugs and they are mostly the forms of Hypokalemic Periodic Paralysis. But, the individuals who take this drug are not without short-term and serious long-term side effects including kidney damage, kidney stones, liver damage, metabolic acidosis, eye issues, bone issues, heart issues, and more. It should not be used by anyone younger than eighteen. It has not been tested on children but is known to affect growth as well as the other mentioned issues.

A majority of individuals who have attempted to use these drugs has had serious effects including comas and sudden death.

To be fair, some individuals do use them with success. Those individuals are extremely lucky, but most still have side effects and need to utilize the natural methods in combination with the drug as well for the best results.

Gather And Share Information

It is important for individuals with Periodic Paralysis to educate themselves and all of those around them. That includes but is not limited to family, friends, neighbors, community, doctors, hospitals, dentist, optometrist and local first responders about every aspect of this condition. Knowing and understanding this medical condition can ease their fears and the fears of those around them and assists with proper management and treatment. Knowing others will be able to provide aid during paralysis episodes is essential.

Join Periodic Paralysis Social Support Groups

Being part of a Periodic Paralysis community is vital. Individuals know they are not alone. One receives encouragement, support, sympathy and empathy and gains information and knowledge from others who live with the same enemy daily. Questions are answered and ideas are shared.

Conclusion

Using the ideas outlined in this part of the chapter, constantly and diligently, day-by-day, minute-by-minute and second-by-second in order to stay balanced may improve the quality of life for individuals in some ways. However, mild, moderate or severe and unpredictable symptoms, periods of paralysis and gradual permanent muscle weakness will more than likely continue to occur in many individuals. How to handle these symptoms and episodes of paralysis when they occur will be covered next.

What Is Periodic Paralysis? A Disease Like No Other

How I reduce and prevent my symptoms:
(You may add your personal information to share with others for their better understanding before you pass along this book.)

Five

Handling The Episodes
Of
Periodic Paralysis

Handling The Symptoms And Paralytic Episodes Once They Begin

When an individual slips into either weakness or paralysis it can be very sudden, without any warning, serious, debilitating and life threatening. It can also be gradual and simply fatiguing. Whatever the case, it can be humiliating, embarrassing, frightening and life changing for the individual who must endure the episode or attack. How this is dealt with can be life saving and face saving or it can harmful and potentially deadly. The individual with Periodic Paralysis needs to know what to do when this happens and must be prepared. His or her family members, friends, teachers, neighbors, co-workers, EMT's, baby-sitters, paramedics, nurses, doctors and more need to know what to do if they are with the person when it happens and must also be prepared.

What Others Can And Must Do To Aide An Individual In An Episode

The following components are more specific for how to treat episodes of weakness or paralysis when they occur for the different forms of Periodic Paralysis. Potassium, whether to take it or not, becomes the main question and concern as an episode begins.

Potassium

For most individuals diagnosed with Periodic Paralysis or with symptoms of Periodic Paralysis, they know or suspect which type they have. As discussed, it is either Hypokalemic Periodic Paralysis, which is low potassium levels, or Hyperkalemic Periodic Paralysis, which are high potassium levels or Normokalemic Periodic Paralysis in which potassium shifts mainly in normal ranges or Andersen-Tawil Syndrome in which any of these may happen.

Using a potassium reader (a very expensive hand-held, non-medical device, which medical insurance will not pay for and is much like a glucose reader for diabetics), can aid in discovering when the level of potassium in blood is too high or too low or within normal ranges. It is best to use the meter to know for sure what the levels are before medicating or taking potassium when symptoms begin. However, symptoms, which typically accompany different levels of potassium for those without a potassium reader, may aid in knowing if the potassium is high or low.

Some individuals with low potassium levels use different types of potassium in a variety of forms. If taken in time, an episode may be stopped or shortened. Their paralysis episodes are fairly well controlled. Others with high potassium do not take potassium, because they already have too much in their systems and this would cause serious paralysis and metabolic acidosis. They can take glucose tablets or eat something with sugar to help control the high amounts of potassium in their blood. Eating carbohydrates or trying to move around, if possible, can also be helpful.

Individuals with Andersen-Tawil-Syndrome or Andersen-Tawil-Syndrome-'like' Periodic Paralysis must be extremely careful when taking potassium. Because, they have periods of high potassium and low potassium, or episodes in normal ranges, it is essential to use a potassium reader to measure the amount in their blood when they begin to feel symptoms or use the list of symptoms to determine the level of potassium. Doing this, will assure that an individual will use the correct method by either taking potassium or eating some carbohydrates or by doing nothing.

Those with symptoms or paralysis while levels of potassium are in normal levels do not need to take potassium. It could cause a rise in potassium levels creating hyperkalemia.

If the episode progresses after this point, the next obvious step is to stop all physical exertion and activity. It may not, however, be a choice for many, who may enter into a total body weakness or full body episode of paralysis.

Cease All Activity

Because, at this point, the muscles become weakened, the ligaments and tendons must take over the work of the muscles. Movement of any type can damage these organs and the muscles more than they are already being damaged. Therefore it is important for the individual to refrain from movement unless it is necessary.

Great care must be used if the individual is to be moved. All weak areas must be well supported.

Provide Comfortable Position

Resting with the head elevated is best for most individuals if on the floor or bed, though some prefer being on their side. Reclining to a comfortable position is usual if sitting. The head easily falls to the left or right due to the weak muscle in the neck and shoulders and this may become very painful. Pillows may be needed to keep the head stable. Hands, arms, feet and legs should be monitored to make sure there is no pinching or cramping.

Provide Comfortable Temperature

Since heat and cold are triggers, it is important that a person does not get too heated under blankets or too chilled without them. He or she should be checked often.

Communicate During An Episode

It is important to communicate during an episode if possible. Many individuals will have some form of information with them about their condition and what to do if they do go into an episode or in an emergency. This may be in the form of a medic alert bracelet, a journal, a grouping of papers with information, a notebook, something worn around the neck, a USB stick, a book like this one or more. Usually, this information is shared ahead of time. How to communicate should be in that information.

Some people are able to communicate during an attack by speaking, but others may have a problem with speech if the muscles in the mouth or the tongue, or both, are affected. Some may be somewhat confused or just too weak. But, if they are able, communication may include blinking for yes or no. Maybe a finger can be moved up for yes and to the side for no. If the head can be moved, perhaps nodding for yes or no will work. So questions should be limited to those that can be answered with a yes or a no. Still others will be in total paralysis with their eyes closed and mouths unable to speak and any communication seems, and may be, impossible.

For them, it is helpful to have patience and to be close, gentle, calm, reassuring and understanding and know that the affected individual can hear everything being said around them and can feel everything done to them. It is important to speak directly to them, explaining what is being done and why it is being done.

Follow Instructions

It is most important to follow the instructions provided, whether planned before an episode or found with the individual at the time of the attack. This can mean the difference between lessening the effects of it and possibly shortening it and it may also mean the difference between life and death for many individuals.

Monitor Vitals

As discussed previously, if at all possible, the vital signs of the individual in an episode need to be monitored. The information should be recorded or written down for future reference. This data is necessary to determine how the person is doing and whether medical assistance may be needed such as a call to the doctor or for an ambulance or for a trip to the ER. Severe issues including heart arrhythmia, breathing, choking or low oxygen, respiratory arrest or cardiac arrest may need immediate help.

If the person is in a full body attack, reporting the vital sign results to them and explaining the details of what is being done is very important. When one cannot see or speak and cannot move in any way, they are extremely vulnerable and usually very stressed and frightened. So speaking to them with all of the information can be very reassuring.

Stay Close

It is prudent to always stay near an individual who is in a paralytic episode. This is for many reasons. Most of these have already been covered. During an episode there are serious medical issues, which can arise. The person is totally vulnerable and not able to do much of anything, if at all, for himself or herself so he or she needs to be closely listened to and observed. Even if she can move, he or she should not. They should be monitored closely, kept comfortable, warm or cool (depending on the situation), and safe.

The medical devices and other necessary items should be close at hand.

Use Of Oxygen During Periods Of Paralysis

Oxygen should be handy to be used for anyone with Periodic Paralysis when in a paralytic episode because very often, an individual develops breathing issues. It can become difficult to breathe and it may feel like an elephant sitting on the chest. Breathing sometimes stops during an episode. Oxygen levels may drop and the person may develop hypoxia or inadequate oxygen levels. This can lead to respiratory arrest and death.

Oxygen should be used for individuals with Andersen-Tawil Syndrome or Andersen-Tawil Syndrome-like symptoms who are in paralytic episodes. An oximeter may not indicate the correct oxygen levels because of chronic or acute dilatation of the heart. This is an enlargement of the heart cavity and death can occur.

Meditation And Mental Imagery

Paralytic attacks can be very frightening and as previously discussed, they may last anywhere from a few minutes to several hours to days at a time. They can involve only parts of the body or the entire body. They may be severe or mild. If and when complications can arise such as breathing problems, heart arrhythmias, muscle cramping or choking, it may be difficult to remain calm.

Learning to relax and just let it happen can be very helpful. Listening to the television or radio, whichever may be on, or the conversations going on among the people around can be reassuring and distracting and a way to keep track of the time. Meditating or using guided imagery can help with relaxation.

There are many websites on the Internet with scripts, audiotapes and videos of guided imagery that can be copied or downloaded for free. These also are available for learning how to meditate.

Conclusion

The most important way for an individual to control and manage the paralytic episodes and other debilitating symptoms is to identify the triggers; substances, activities, foods or more, which are causing them and then to avoid them. Equally important is maintaining 'balance' in all aspects of life for individuals with Periodic Paralysis. With these methods some control may be regained in life by reducing the number and severity of the paralytic episodes and other symptoms and the debilitating complications experienced. Following the ideas, which use natural methods and common sense ideas, the cruel symptoms of Periodic Paralysis will be relieved in some ways for everyone who seriously attempts to stay balanced and can 'be the best they can be naturally.'

That being said, however, many individuals can follow all of these ideas and methods and still have severe and unpredictable symptoms, episodes of paralysis, gradual permanent muscle weakness and continue to be very ill, debilitated and disabled. This may be due to many reasons, such as the type of Periodic Paralysis, co-existing conditions, previous damage done due to a lack of diagnosis and proper treatment and inappropriate drugs prescribed. Most people will also eventually need the use of assistive and adaptive technology such as canes, crutches, wheelchairs and power wheelchairs and they will need the aid of family members and caregivers.

Although most episodes of weakness and paralysis are frightening, especially in the beginning, most individuals will learn that once an episode begins, the best and only thing one can do is to stay calm and try to relax. However, it is best to have a caregiver close in order to monitor the vitals. If there is choking, heart arrhythmia, extreme blood pressure or heart rate or if breathing stops, then it may be necessary to call for emergency care.

The help I need during an episode:
(You may add your personal information to share with others for their better understanding before you pass along this book.)

Handling The Episodes Of Periodic Paralysis

Six

Diagnosing Periodic Paralysis

Periodic Paralysis Takes An Average Of Twenty Years To Diagnose

Receiving a diagnosing for Periodic Paralysis is very difficult in many cases. Although unbelievable, but true, it takes an average of twenty years to be diagnosed with most forms of Periodic Paralysis! This is a very serious issue because the earlier a diagnosis is made and proper treatment has begun, the better the chance for a more positive and better outcome.

Some individuals are in their sixth and seventh decade before finally receiving a diagnosis; others live their entire lives without knowing what had been plaguing them throughout their lifetime and still others die before getting a diagnosis due to the lack of diagnosis and improper treatment. There are even more individuals who are misdiagnosed, mistreated with improper or unnecessary drugs and harmed for the remainder of their lives. Many are humiliated and misdiagnosed with mental disorders, such as hypochondria and 'conversion disorder.'

The reasons are many, but the most obvious is that it is unrecognized by medical professionals. Only a paragraph or two is devoted to it in medical school texts and it is explained that doctors will probably never see anyone with it. Another reason is that most of the information, which does exist, is outdated and for the most part wrong, and only involves Hypokalemic Periodic Paralysis, which involves only low potassium and full-body paralysis. Other forms and atypical symptoms are dismissed. One more important reason is, unfortunately, Periodic Paralysis is diagnosed after all else has been ruled out. That involves many years of testing and frustration.

How Periodic Paralysis Is Diagnosed

There are two methods used for diagnosis of the various types of Periodic Paralysis; one is through genetic testing, which studies one's DNA. If a mutation is found the person receives a 'genetic' diagnosis. The following are the known genetic mutations for the forms of Periodic Paralysis.

Criteria For Making A Genetic Diagnosis

Hypokalemic Periodic Paralysis is caused by abnormalities in the SCN4A, KCNJ18 and CACNA1S genes.

Hyperkalemic Periodic Paralysis is caused by abnormalities in the SCN4A gene.

Andersen-Tawil Syndrome is caused by abnormalities in the KCNJ2 gene and the KCNJ5 gene.

Normokalemic Periodic Paralysis is caused by abnormalities in the SCN4A and CACNA1C genes.

Paramyotonia Congenita is caused by abnormalities in the SCN4A gene.

Thyrotoxic Periodic Paralysis is caused by abnormalities in the KCNE3 and KCNJ18 genes.

My known genetic marker is:
(You may add your personal information to share with others for their better understanding before you pass along this book.)

Problems With Genetic Testing

Although genetic or DNA testing is available, it is extremely expensive and most medical insurance companies will not pay for it. It is also biased, limited and narrow and will locate less than one half of the genetic markers, abnormalities or mutations. This is due to the fact that about fifty percent of the mutations for the various forms of Periodic Paralysis are not known and have not actually been discovered yet and when testing is ordered, not all forms, which are known, are selected to be searched for in the testing. Most doctors will only order testing for Hypokalemic Periodic Paralysis. This means that DNA testing has much less than a fifty percent chance of locating a genetic marker for an individual for a Periodic Paralysis diagnosis.

Most medical professionals and doctors do not know about or understand this. So, if and when, the test results are negative, most medical professionals will not diagnose with Periodic Paralysis, but instead diagnose with a mental or functional condition or with another harmful misdiagnosis.

Due to these issues, Periodic Paralysis needs to be diagnosed clinically.

The Clinical Diagnosis

If a person is diagnosed based on his or her symptoms and characteristics, once all else has been ruled out, it is called a 'clinical' diagnosis. This can and may be simple and easy for those who may have forms of Hypokalemic Periodic Paralysis. If an individual has consistently low potassium levels combined with obvious episodes of paralysis, a diagnosis can be made quickly. The same would be for those with some forms of Hyperkalemic Periodic Paralysis. If an individual has consistently high potassium levels combined with obvious episodes of paralysis, a diagnosis can also be made quickly. Other forms of this condition are not as clear-cut due to all of the symptoms, which may occur as discussed previously. Potassium levels may remain in normal ranges, or they may sometimes be low, high or in normal ranges with symptoms, coexisting conditions may exist, inappropriate drugs prescribed may cause new symptoms or change previous ones.

Because the symptoms look neurological, patients will typically be sent to neurologists. Unfortunately, this will begin the cycle of years of testing, drugs being prescribed for neurological conditions, which do not exist, more and different symptoms develop, more wrong diagnoses are made, and more harm is done. An individual becomes stuck in the 'diagnosis dilemma.' This is a serious situation because those with Periodic Paralysis need to have a diagnosis.

The Reasons A Diagnosis Is Necessary

Individuals with Periodic Paralysis need a diagnosis for many reasons. It is needed for safety reasons in the doctors' office, the dentist office, an ambulance ride, the ER, the hospital, for surgeries and in any emergency. Most cannot take any drugs or medications due to idiosyncratic, paradoxical and iatrogenic effects nor can they have IV's because sodium and glucose can shift the potassium even lower and causes other life-threatening symptoms nor can they tolerate anesthesia due to possible malignant hyperthermia and/or more paralysis, life-threatening heart arrhythmia, possible cessation of breathing and death. A diagnosis is necessary because people with Periodic Paralysis need to be safe and free from harm in any and all situations.

The medical professionals need to know that a patient has Periodic Paralysis and how to treat or not treat him or her, as the case may be. They need to know that when a person is in paralysis and struggling with arrhythmia, fluctuating blood pressure and heart rate, choking, breathing issues and pain, that although they cannot open their eyes or speak, they can hear everything going on around them. They need to know that the person is not faking nor making it up. Does a doctor really think that someone wants to be totally helpless and struggling for his or her life?

A diagnosis is also needed to stop the constant, expensive and insane cycle of testing and retesting for every condition under the sun for an average of twenty years out of a person's life. How many medical conditions exist in which an individual intermittently has episodes of paralysis?

During the cycle of insanity for a diagnosis, drugs of every type are prescribed which are unnecessary and harmful causing more damage and possible death. New symptoms may develop and then more testing is done and new drugs prescribed. The insanity continues. Then comes the diagnosis of 'conversion disorder' or 'somatic symptoms.' Psychotropic drugs are prescribed at this point. More damage is done and possible death may occur.

Without a diagnosis and proper treatment, the individual naturally becomes more ill because organs in the body are being damaged from the potassium shifting, exercise intolerance and gradual permanent muscle weakness sets in, heart problems get more severe, breathing muscles become affected, kidney stones develop, osteoporosis, metabolic acidosis can cause death. Adaptive equipment like power wheelchairs and oxygen may be necessary. Without a diagnosis the patients will be unable to receive these much needed aides. Without a diagnosis, disability or social security is impossible to receive.

The child, teenager and young adult with Periodic Paralysis will need a diagnosis for appropriate treatment. He or she will need accommodations in school. Teachers, coaches and school nurses need to know how to deal with the symptoms and paralysis and understand what is happening and why. There may be a great deal of school missed. Sports and other activities need to be avoided. A special diet must be followed. Wheelchairs or other adaptive equipment may be needed. Without a diagnosis none of this will happen.

For the adult trying to support a family by holding down a job or a career and living with Periodic Paralysis without a diagnosis and proper treatment may lose their job. The years and years of medical testing, misdiagnosis, inappropriate treatment wrong medications, and more can result in financial ruin. This can lead to homes being lost, divorce may ensue, families will fall apart, friends back away, depression sets in and possible suicide may occur. A clear diagnosis and treatment may help others like employers, family members and friends to understand and be willing to help. Disability may be possible.

One of the most important results of a diagnosis for the individual with Periodic Paralysis and his or her family is validation. Validation that the illness does truly exist and that he or she is finally believed. They are vindicated. Vindicated of making it up, faking it or being a hypochondriac. They do not have 'conversion disorder.' They have been telling the truth.

The Clinical Diagnosis

'Hit them between the eyes with the facts.'

Because a diagnosis is so difficult to obtain, it is important for the individual who believes he or she has a form of Periodic Paralysis to take the lead to basically diagnose himself or herself and then to become his or her own team leader in order to get a diagnosis from a doctor.

The best way to get a clinical diagnosis is to gather as much information together as possible to prove one's case. Once all of the information is gathered, an individual can 'Hit them (the doctors) between the eyes with the facts.' This is done by videotaping the episodes, keeping a journal and putting together a notebook with all of the testing results and more. Things that need to be included are ER visit reports, hospital records, doctors' notes, records of the vitals, and more, depending on one's symptoms and one's particular case. (Two books previously written and published by the Periodic Paralysis Network contain charts, forms and more to use for this purpose, including the instructions.)

The following outline has aided individuals to obtain a diagnosis. It takes a great deal of time and work for one who is so very ill, but with very few doctors who understand this rare condition, there is not much of a choice. It is up to the patient, hopefully with the aid of family and friends, to put it all together.

The following plan illustrates the complexity and the obvious time and costs involved in obtaining a diagnosis of Periodic Paralysis. It should not be this difficult for anyone to get a diagnosis for any disease.

The Diagnosis Plan

Gathering The Facts:

One must **gather the facts**. It is important for **everything else to be ruled out**. A Primary Care Physician (PCP) and a neurologist normally do this, because most of the symptoms resemble neuromuscular disorders. The tests ruling everything else out might include but are not limited to:
- Lab work of all types,
  - Blood
  - Urine
- MRI's,
  - Brain
  - Spine
- Spinal taps,
- X-rays
- EEGs
- EMGs
- EKGs
- CMAPs
- Muscle biopsy

(Some of the tests above may show changes that can be markers for PP).

Most doctors diagnosing Periodic Paralysis want lab work showing either:
- Paralysis during shifting in normal ranges
- Paralysis during shifting in low potassium and/or,
- Paralysis during shifting high potassium
  - This is done by obtaining blood potassium levels
    - May need to be done several times until a baseline is established.

- Then during episodes every 5 to 10 minutes...not just one blood draw...there is no way to see the shifting otherwise.
- It may be necessary for hospitalization in order to do this while in the paralysis.
- It may need to be done for more than 24 hours until each is documented, during the episodes.
- If the shifting is in the normal ranges, it may never show up during tests, unless it is done every few minutes.
  - More than 50% of PP patients may not have potassium shifting out of normal ranges.
  - ATS patients may shift all three ways.
- However, the latest information for diagnosing PP based on potassium levels in blood serum is as follows:
  - The potassium in the blood does not always shift above or below normal ranges in 50% or more of patients experiencing muscle weakness or paralysis or it shifts so quickly that it cannot be measured. Doctors need to diagnose a patient with Periodic Paralysis based on his or her symptoms, specifically, heart symptoms on an EKG and the muscle strength or weakness and history of episodes of paralysis.
- ** The information above needs to be shared with the doctors. Most do not understand these concepts. **

❖ There needs to be periods of paralysis, either total or partial, or muscle weakness, which can be documented (or gradual, progressive, fixed muscle weakness; all other things ruled out).
- Videotaping is the best way to do this.
- It may be necessary for hospitalization in order for doctors to see an individual while paralyzed

or with periods of weak muscles.

Warning!

Under no circumstances, for the purpose of trying to get a diagnosis, should an individual provoke his or her symptoms or an episode of paralysis by omitting medication or ingesting drugs, or foods or perform activities, which are known triggers. This is a very serious thing to do. Many doctors attempt to have their patients do this for an easy diagnosis. Some individuals have done this and it has led to their death.

- ECGs or EKGs consistent with 'ion channelopathy,' Periodic Paralysis or Andersen-Tawil Syndrome.
    - Needs to be done while in the paralysis, so it may need to be done for more than 24 hours until each is documented, during an episode.
        - Holter Heart Monitors are best for this.
- Oximeter (oxygen) recordings:
    - Indicating, levels dropping during paralysis.
    - If in an advanced case of PP, it may show hypoventilation.
- Gather all previous medical records.
    - Obtain all doctors' records from each appointment attended.
    - Obtain copies of all lab records, x-rays, hospitalizations, and more.
- Chart the triggers for the episodes.
- Document an increase of episodes after eating carbohydrates, sugar, salt or red meat, after exercising or after taking certain medications. This is important for being able to control the

episodes and allowing the doctors to know what the triggers are to aid in a diagnosis.
- ❖ Document a reduction of episodes when using potassium is good. This can indicate the loss of potassium after shifting and may indicate low potassium levels.
- ❖ Gather a team of doctors. (Knowledgeable about PP or willing to learn)
  - ➢ PCP
  - ➢ Neurologist
  - ➢ Electrocardiologist
  - ➢ Nephrologist
  - ➢ Endocrinologist
  - ➢ Counselor or therapist
  - ➢ Others as needed for symptoms
  - ➢ MDA doctors who understand Periodic Paralysis if possible
- ❖ Gather as much medical information as possible from family members who may have symptoms similar to Periodic Paralysis. It has a hereditary component.
- ❖ If one suspects Andersen-Tawil Syndrome, gather as much medical information as possible from family members and note the symptoms and characteristics. Create a family flowchart with this information. Adding pictures can be helpful in demonstrating the characteristics.

It seems that doctors need better, more thorough and up-to-date training of this complex, misunderstood and rare mineral metabolic disorder for timelier recognition, diagnosis and treatment. The sooner an individual receives a diagnosis; the better chance there is for a more positive outcome in many ways.

My diagnosis took _____ years.
(You may add your personal information to share with others for their better understanding before you pass along this book.)

The type of diagnosis I have is:

I have been seeking a diagnosis for _____ years.

Seven

Complications Of Periodic Paralysis

Possible Complications

The Most Common

There is no doubt that many complications are associated with Periodic Paralysis, especially when the condition has been misdiagnosed and mistreated over many years. The following are some of the more common complications found in many individuals with all forms of Periodic Paralysis.

Progressive Permanent Muscle Weakness (PMW)

In Periodic Paralysis there is generalized weakness, because the muscles of the entire body are involved. There is no loss of sensation or feeling, however. The weakness is usually most noticeable in what are called the proximal muscles, those closest to the trunk, and the largest of the muscle groups. The weakness is equal on both sides of the body. And, although the weakness and paralysis are intermittent and have a beginning and an end in most cases, for some the weakness becomes chronic, or occurring over a long span of time or it returns often. The chronic weakness can become slowly progressive and fixed or permanent. Once it becomes chronic it can cause muscle wasting and fat or lipid can replace the muscle. At the point the muscle weakness becomes permanent, it will not go away and at this point it is progressive meaning it will steadily continue to worsen.

Exercise Intolerance

In exercise intolerance the individual is not able to do physical exercise or exertion that would be expected from someone of his or her age and overall health level nor for the amount of time expected. He or she lacks stamina. The individual may also experience extreme pain and fatigue after exercising or exertion and other symptoms such as a feeling of heaviness in the muscle groups.

Food and oxygen are normally converted into energy and delivered to the muscles but this cycle is disrupted in individuals with exercise intolerance. The muscles are unable to use the nutrients and oxygen and therefore, enough energy may not be generated to the muscles and he or she is left with little or no energy. The degrees of low energy can be mild or extreme and the symptoms may occur during exercise or exertion or they can occur later, even the next day.

Heart Issues

Abnormal heart rhythms are serious and life-threatening complications for individuals with Periodic Paralysis. Each of the three forms, Hypokalemic Periodic Paralysis, Hyperkalemic Periodic Paralysis and Anderson-Tawil Syndrome, has a specific pattern of irregular heartbeats, which makes it easy to identify on an electrical study of the heart called an electrocardiogram (EKG). It is not necessary to explain or understand each irregular heartbeat or pattern. They are however, referenced in the following sections for recognition and for diagnosis by physicians and patients.

Hypokalemic Periodic Paralysis

When an individual with Periodic Paralysis begins to experience a decrease in potassium, there is a decrease in the 'T' wave. The next step is an 'ST-segment depression' and then the 'T' waves become inverted or 'flip.' At the same time the 'PR' interval becomes prolonged and the 'P' wave enlarges. A 'U' wave appears after the 'T' wave and can be seen on the mid-precordial leads. When the 'U' wave becomes larger than the 'T' wave develops on the EKG, the potassium level in less than 3 (<3). As the potassium levels decrease further, the 'T' and 'U' wave combine into a prominent 'U' wave on the EKG. This makes the 'T' waves visible.

At this point, in severe hypokalemia, a person might also develop ventricular tachycardia (fast heart beat) and/or ventricular fibrillation. The fibers of the ventricle of the heart contract in an uncontrolled and random manner. When this happens, without immediate medical help, the individual will die because the heart can stop beating suddenly and unexpectedly from cardiac arrest. Occasionally atrioventricular block, which is a sudden pause or bradycardia that is a slow heartbeat (under 60 beats per minute) can occur. So, in episodes of hypokalemia in individuals with Periodic Paralysis, there may be either a fast heartbeat or a slow heartbeat along with the specific arrhythmia.

Hyperkalemic Periodic Paralysis

If an individual has mild to moderately high potassium levels in his or her blood, 'P' wave becomes smaller in size and a peaked 'T' wave develops on an electrocardiogram (EKG). In more dangerous higher levels of potassium it affects the electrical conduction of the heart in the sinoatrial (SA) of the heart. The SA is the 'pacemaker' of the heart and responsible for the contraction of a heart beat.

On an EKG the 'P' wave disappears and the ventricular contraction lengthens. This appears on an EKG as a 'QRS complex'. The overall pumping of the heart decreases to below 60 beats per minute and this is called bradycardia. The pulse becomes weak and heart block may occur. There may also be an increase in the heart rate called ventricular tachycardia. Arrhythmias in the form of ventricular fibrillation may also occur. So, in episodes of hyperkalemia in individuals with Periodic Paralysis, there may be either a fast heartbeat or a slow heartbeat along with the specific arrhythmia.

Andersen-Tawil Syndrome

In an individual with Andersen-Tawil Syndrome, the heart complications are very distinctive, extremely serious and some of the arrhythmias are life threatening. They can include prominent two-phased 'U' waves, down sloped terminal 'T' waves which are prolonged, wide 'TU' waves, premature ventricular complexes (PVCs), ventricular arrhythmias, including ventricular tachycardia, ventricular tachycardia which is bidirectional (BVT), supraventricular tachycardia, ventricular fibrillation, long QT interval heart beat (a ventricular tachycardia) and torsades de pointes.

He or she may have no symptoms although they are experiencing arrhythmias, or they may have minor symptoms despite experiencing a serious number of arrhythmias and tachycardia or they may be very symptomatic. Regardless of the symptoms, a person is at high-risk for sudden death from an arrhythmia, namely the long QT heartbeat (LQT), the torsades de pointes and the ventricular fibrillation.

The changes, which are most common and affect the heart most often in Andersen-Tawil

Syndrome, are the ventricular arrhythmias. This is a disruption in the lower chambers of the heart. In the long QT heart beat the heart muscle takes longer than normal between beats to recharge. When this condition is not treated it leads to uncomfortable feelings, syncope, (fainting) or cardiac arrest. The long QT interval heartbeat is one of the distinguishing features used to identify and diagnose Andersen-Tawil Syndrome.

There may be no actual, underlying cardiac disease in individuals with Andersen-Tawil Syndrome, but rather they are born with the predisposition to develop, under certain circumstances (triggers), the ventricular tachycardia and arrhythmias identified here. However, cardiomyopathy, a disease of the heart muscle, often develops in persons with Anderson-Tawil Syndrome. The heart becomes thickened and/or enlarged and weakens. This leads to heart failure.

The Need For Oxygen

The potassium shifting and depletion that occurs in Periodic Paralysis can affect all the muscles of the body including the heart muscle and the respiratory (breathing) muscles. The muscles can become permanently weakened and this includes the heart and breathing muscles. This weakness of the heart muscle and breathing muscles can be fatal in Periodic Paralysis. The diaphragm is the primary breathing muscle. The intercostal muscles are secondary breathing muscles. Breathing involves all the muscles from mouth to lower abdomen. Paralysis of the diaphragm can cause respiratory arrest or the sudden stoppage of breathing.

If the organs are deprived of oxygen, the heart and the rest of the body are working harder to stay alive. This can cause an individual with PP to develop hypoventilation. This is a condition in which one is barely breathing due to weak breathing muscles which prompts him or her to breath less and less over time. Eventually one will get accustomed to getting by on less oxygen while excess carbon dioxide is stored in his muscles and organs. This can cause long-term problems including damage to most of the organs and muscles in the body, but the heart and brain are particularly vulnerable. Oxygen therapy may be necessary at this point.

Kidney Issues

Kidney function can be affected in individuals with Periodic Paralysis. We know that when potassium shifts, calcium carbonate from the bone is released. This increase of calcium carbonate, can lead to the formation of kidney stones. We also know if one has chronic metabolic acidosis, as a result of Periodic Paralysis, his or her kidneys can be affected because metabolic acidosis also causes an increase or shifting of potassium into the body fluids causing an increase of calcium carbonate. The use of the commonly used diuretic for patients with Periodic Paralysis, acetazolamide, also known as diamox, can cause kidney stones.

Osteoporosis

When potassium shifts in the body, as it does in Periodic Paralysis, calcium carbonate from the bone is released. This causes a loss of the bone crystals in the bones leading to osteoporosis. Chronic metabolic acidosis, as a result of Periodic Paralysis, also causes the potassium to shift, thus creating bone loss or osteoporosis.

Research indicates there is a connection between Periodic Paralysis and the osteoporosis. Some individuals with Periodic Paralysis can develop early bone loss due to the potassium shifting out of the bones and other organs as it shifts into the muscles. During the shifting, there is a loss of the bone crystals causing bone-loss or osteoporosis.

Metabolic Acidosis/Lactic Acidosis

Metabolic acidosis and lactic acidosis are complex conditions, which can be difficult to understand, but fairly easy to diagnose based on symptoms and lab results. However, in individuals with Periodic Paralysis, they are often overlooked, missed on the lab reports and testing for them is often not requested as a possibility for obvious symptoms. Because Periodic Paralysis is a mineral metabolic disorder and it affects the breathing muscles, individuals with it appear to be susceptible for developing these conditions. Episodes of paralysis are triggered by metabolic and lactic acidosis.

Metabolic acidosis is a pH imbalance (the balance between the acid and alkaline), in which the body accumulates an excess of acid in the body fluids and does not have enough bicarbonate to neutralize the effects of the acid effectively. An individual can develop metabolic acidosis, if the carbon dioxide levels are allowed to rise and remain in the body.

Metabolic acidosis affects the heart and breathing. It results in potassium shifting out of the cells and into the bloodstream creating hyperkalemia, too much potassium. The combination of metabolic acidosis and hyperkalemia is a serious condition and can be life threatening leading to shock and death.

In chronic metabolic acidosis an individual's bones and kidneys are affected. When potassium shifts in the body, calcium carbonate from the bone is released. This causes a loss of the bone crystals leading to osteoporosis. When the kidneys are affected, this can be seen by the formation of kidney stones.

Lactic Acidosis

Lactic acidosis is a form of metabolic acidosis that occurs when blood pH levels in the blood and lactic acid become unbalanced. This is the result of oxygen levels dropping. It forms if the carbohydrates get broken down and are used for energy from the low oxygen levels. The lactic acid increases in the bloodstream more quickly than it can be expelled. Too much lactic acid in the body creates an increase of pyruvic acid. Too much pyruvic acid in the body creates metabolic acid in the body. It can cause mental confusion and lead to a coma. It affects the function of the liver and can develop into multiple organ failure, which can lead to death.

Lactic acidosis can develop in individuals with metabolic disorders, especially ones that do not supply enough oxygen to tissues in the body. This kind is known as Type A lactic acidosis. Because Periodic Paralysis is a disorder in which hypoventilation (slow and shallow breathing) can occur when the breathing muscles weaken, individuals with it, can and do develop metabolic and lactic acidosis.

Lactic acidosis is an indication that there may be mitochondrial damage in the cells from the continual potassium shifting from Periodic Paralysis. This damage of the mitochondria may lead to issues of the autoimmune system leading to autoimmune dysfunction, disorders and diseases.

Pain

Unfortunately, many doctors have the misconception, based on outdated and archaic information and data, that pain is a not a symptom and does not exist in patients who have Periodic Paralysis. This is a serious issue because these doctors refuse to recognize Periodic Paralysis and refuse to diagnose individuals who desperately need to be diagnosed if they experience pain.

Surveys indicate that about ninety-five percent of individuals with Periodic Paralysis, regardless of their diagnoses; Andersen-Tawil Syndrome, Hypokalemic Periodic Paralysis, Hyperkalemic Periodic Paralysis, Normokalemic Periodic Paralysis or Paramyotonia Congenita experience pain.

The pain can be experienced before, at the beginning; during or after episodes or it can be intermittent or chronic (all of the time). The pain was described in many ways such as achy, sharp, constant, tenderness, sudden, cramping, rigidity, contractions, tightening, stiffness, charley horses, growing pains or spasms. It was reported as only involving one limb or body part, partial body, the trunk, several body parts or the entire body.

The pain results from several natural ways depending on the type of Periodic Paralysis or genetic mutation. In some cases it is from the swelling of the muscles when they fill up with fluid as the potassium shifts. Some of the pain is from the rigidity and contracting of the muscles. A third cause can be the shifting of sugar with the potassium. A fourth cause may be from low magnesium. Cold can create rigidity and pain for some. Metabolic acidosis, which can often develop in Periodic Paralysis, causes pain in the bones and chest pain.

Other conditions or diseases can co-exist causing permanent or intermittent pain such as Ehlers-Danlos Syndrome (EDS), fibromyalgia or arthritis. These may be aggravated when an individual with Periodic Paralysis is in an episode or paralysis. Intermittent paralytic episodes can damage organs in the body, including the muscles. For some individuals the pain becomes permanent and may be misdiagnosed as fibromyalgia, or other medical issues like rheumatoid arthritis. Pain may also be caused from other unnatural means. The off-label medications typically prescribed for Periodic Paralysis or other drugs such as statins may create pain.

Rhabdomyolysis

Rhabdomyolysis, or muscle wasting, is a serious condition, which is seen in some forms of Periodic Paralysis. It can be caused from low potassium levels. Those with Hypokalemic Periodic Paralysis, especially mutations found in CACNA1S, seem to be more likely to develop it.

In Rhabdomyolysis, skeletal muscle breaks down very quickly. The particles of the damaged muscle enter the bloodstream and are harmful to the kidneys and may cause kidney failure. The symptoms from this can be quite severe including vomiting, pain in the muscles, arrhythmia, tachycardia, confusion and even coma. The more severe the muscle damage, the more serious the symptoms become. Tea-colored urine may develop.

Drugs and Medications

Paradoxical Reaction And Idiosyncratic Reaction To Drugs

As mentioned previously, the two most common issues with drugs or pharmaceuticals for individuals with Periodic Paralysis (and others) are a paradoxical reaction and an idiosyncratic reaction. These are both serious effects. If one has a paradoxical reaction to a medication it means that the opposite of what is supposed to happen will occur. For instance, if someone takes a sleeping pill and then stays awake all night, it is known as a paradoxical effect. This can be just an inconvenience or very serious depending on the medical issue and the reaction. If someone who is already experiencing high blood pressure, is prescribed a drug to lower blood pressure, but it increases the blood pressure, this can cause a stroke, other serious effects or even death.

If an individual develops tremors, metabolic acidosis and paralysis from taking an antibiotic; these would be considered as idiosyncratic effects, reactions or side effects, which would be totally unpredicted, unexpected and never seen before. These effects would not already be listed as possible rare side effects. This is a serious problem because these idiosyncratic effects, also known as 'type B reaction,' can be harmful by causing damage or even death. The amount ingested has no bearing on it. The reactions may occur from the smallest amount possible after one dose and the reactions may occur right away or after a little passage of time, even after a few weeks or chronically after a period of time.

Research indicates idiosyncratic effects are related to metabolic, mitochondrial and inflammatory dysfunction rather than the immune system and that there might be a genetic link in many cases.

Why is this an issue for individuals with Periodic Paralysis? Periodic Paralysis is a mineral metabolic disorder. Paradoxical reactions and idiosyncratic reactions are related to metabolic dysfunction. Strange, odd and out of the ordinary side effects and drugs creating the opposite effects are common characteristics of individuals with all forms of Periodic Paralysis, especially the form known as Andersen-Tawil Syndrome.

Many individuals with Periodic Paralysis have serious side effects from the drugs they are prescribed. Without knowing this and without a diagnosis, doctors will prescribe drugs to treat symptoms that appear to be neurological or for other issues. The patient will use the pharmaceuticals and develop new symptoms, over time. These symptoms begin to look like something else for which new medications are prescribed, and the cycle continues. Or if there is no diagnosis and a person is suspected of having a conversion disorder, once everything else is ruled out, psychotropic medications may be prescribed. These medications can become out of control and it is not uncommon to be on 5 or 10 or more drugs at one time. They are toxic to the body and are causing damage. Most of them are also triggers for the periods of paralysis, and each paralytic episode causes more damage to the body.

In conclusion, a paradoxical or idiosyncratic reaction is an immune system response to drugs due to genetic predisposition and metabolic dysfunction in individuals with Periodic Paralysis, a mineral metabolic disorder. This includes the medications specifically prescribed to treat Periodic Paralysis. Precautions must be taken to avoid these effects.

Acetazolamide-Diamox

One of the major drugs used for treating Periodic Paralysis is acetazolamide, also sold under the name of diamox. It is an off-label drug, which means this drug is made and used to treat conditions other than Periodic Paralysis. It is a carbonic anhydrase inhibitor, which is a diuretic. It removes water through the kidneys. Interestingly, it is used to treat mild metabolic acidosis (discussed above), however, it actually leads to more metabolic acidosis by speeding up the process. Many individuals taking this drug to treat their symptoms of Periodic Paralysis are unknowingly making themselves worse and causing more damage to their bodies. It also lowers potassium so it is questionable for use with Hypokalemic Periodic Paralysis. It is also linked to permanent muscle weakness. Many people are also unaware that it is a sulfa-based drug and should not be taken if an allergy exists to sulfa drugs.

If one already has Periodic Paralysis and has chronic metabolic acidosis, he or she can develop kidney stones and osteoporosis over time. If one already has Periodic Paralysis and has chronic metabolic acidosis and takes diamox, he or she can become more acidic and can acquire full blown metabolic acidosis which causes more damage and kidney stones and accelerates osteoporosis, more illness, more paralysis from the stress on the body and lowering of potassium and may even cause death.

There are also warnings about children using acetazolamide. The safety and effectiveness have not even been tested for those under twelve. There are three major side effects seen in children; 'fits,' growth retardation and weakening of the bones.

Research indicates that only 50% of those with Hypokalemic Periodic Paralysis, especially with the SCN4A genetic mutation, do not respond to acetazolamide and it may actually cause paralysis or worse symptoms. So, if someone is diagnosed with Hypokalemic Periodic Paralysis, they must be very careful, it should be used with extreme caution. It should not automatically be given to people who are clinically diagnosed with Hypokalemic Periodic Paralysis or if it is, it should be monitored closely.

About half of the individuals with Periodic Paralysis do not have a genetic diagnosis and do not know what sequence or genetic mutation they actually have. Further study and research are recommended before taking it so one will know what to expect or what to look for, in order to be safe.

Some do well on this medication. If it is working and there are no side effects, then there are no problems. If, however, this drug may be causing side effects or if one is attempting to decide whether to take it or not, hopefully this information can help in making an informed decision.

Intravenous Therapy (IV's)

One of the greatest fears individuals with Periodic Paralysis have is ending up in the ER at the mercy of doctors who do not understand the condition while they are in full body paralysis. The first thing medical professionals want to do is attach an IV, short for intravenous therapy. This is frightening because they can be a serious trigger for most forms of Periodic Paralysis. IV's of glucose or dextrose (sugar and water), or saline or sodium (salt and water) can create paralysis; make an episode worse and in some cases cause death.

If an IV is needed in an emergency situation, for severely low potassium, mannitol may be used in diluted strengths and only small amounts every twenty to sixty minutes. Hyperkalemia may develop otherwise. Close monitoring of the heart and potassium levels are necessary. It must be used with great care because it is also dehydrating.

Individuals with Hyperkalemic Periodic Paralysis may benefit from the use of a glucose IV.

Individuals with Periodic Paralysis have used Hartmann's IV Solution with some success. It may be a good option, especially if acidosis is present. It contains a mixture of electrolytes.

Many individuals with Periodic Paralysis are made to endure pain, more paralysis, harm and sometimes-even death due to doctors not listening to the patients or their family members about this serious issue.

Anesthesia

As previously discussed, Periodic Paralysis is an ion channelopathy, which is a dysfunction of the ion channels. The ion channels transport the electrolytes, such as sodium and potassium through the cells. This transport is faulty in individuals with ion channel dysfunction and extreme care must be used when anesthesia is going to be utilized. This is due to the possibility of developing serious symptoms such as breathing issues or failure, arrhythmia, blood pressure issues, choking, muscle weakness or paralysis, longer recovery after surgery, malignant hyperthermia or death. Managing the use of anesthesia in individuals with Periodic Paralysis is mostly aimed at preventing attacks of paralysis or the other symptoms during or after surgery. The manner in which the situation is handled for the individual depends on which form of Periodic Paralysis is involved.

Malignant Hyperthermia (MH): As mentioned previously, individuals with Periodic Paralysis are at risk for developing malignant hyperthermia during or after surgery. Many forms of Periodic Paralysis are the result of mutations on Chromosome 17. Malignant hyperthermia is also the result of a mutation on Chromosome 17, thus creating the potential for those with Periodic Paralysis, including, Normokalemic Periodic Paralysis, to develop the serious and life-threatening symptoms involved with the use of anesthesia.

Hypokalemic Periodic Paralysis and Anesthesia: For individuals with Hypokalemic Periodic Paralysis, anesthesia is a known trigger for paralytic episodes. According to research, in order to successfully manage the patient there is need for an evaluation before surgery, avoidance of known triggers, careful monitoring during the surgery and immediate and proper treatment if an issue arises.

Hyperkalemic Periodic Paralysis and Anesthesia: Nothing was written about the use of anesthesia and Hyperkalemic Periodic Paralysis before 2002. Early research concluded that anesthesia might be used without complications if the potassium levels were within normal levels prior to surgery, if the carbohydrate levels were up, if anesthetic drugs, which released potassium, were not used and if normal body temperature levels were maintained.

Andersen-Tawil Syndrome and Anesthesia: Some research indicated that malignant hyperthermia is not usually an issue for individuals with Andersen-Tawil Syndrome. However, it is an issue because individuals with ATS have shifting of potassium into both high and low ranges causing symptoms and paralysis. The other issue with anesthesia use and ATS is a need for special precautions due to the serious issue of the long QT interval heartbeat, a diagnostic marker for the condition and torsades de pointes another extremely serious arrhythmia. There are many medications that must be avoided, which are used routinely in preparation for surgery and during surgery including the glucose and sodium IVs, as well as most forms of anesthesia.

Lidocaine: Topical, regional and local anesthesia may cause potassium to drop in individuals with Hypokalemic Periodic Paralysis, Normokalemic Periodic Paralysis or Andersen-Tawil Syndrome if it contains epinephrine. The most often discussed and utilized local anesthesia is lidocaine. For some individuals it may work well if the epinephrine is removed. For others it may cause hypokalemia or arrhythmia regardless of the epinephrine being removed. For others still, it may not work at all or the usual amount may be needed during a procedure. Lidocaine and other local types of anesthesia need to be used with extreme caution.

Anyone with Periodic Paralysis needs to be extremely cautious when planning any surgical procedures, which may use anesthesia.

No Tourniquet

Another complication that needs to be included here is related to the drawing of blood for measuring potassium levels in the blood. It is recommended that a tourniquet should not be used. When blood is drawn using a tourniquet it can result in potassium levels, which are higher than they really are. It is important to understand that improper use of a tourniquet and the clenching of the fist can result in false lab results for potassium levels. The pressure (too tight) and time (too long) of the tourniquet can raise the level of potassium as much as 10% to 20%. This difference can be important when making a decision about treatment or trying to get diagnosed.

As explained at the beginning of this chapter, many complications are associated with Periodic Paralysis, especially when the condition has been misdiagnosed and mistreated over a period of many years. The next section will discuss more complex issues and obstacles related to this condition.

My common complications:
(You may add your personal information to share with others for their better understanding before you pass along this book.)

More Complications

Understanding The Complexity

Several other forms of complications, confusion, difficulty and obstacles exist for recognition, diagnosis and treatment related to Periodic Paralysis. These are more complex and multifaceted than those discussed previously. They are serious, seldom discussed and most certainly overlooked.

Co-Existing Conditions

The term 'co-existing conditions' also known as 'co-morbidity' means having more than one medical condition, illness or disease at the same time. Many individuals diagnosed with a form of Periodic Paralysis have at least one more other diagnosed condition. Most have, and a few had as many as fifteen other diagnosed diseases, conditions or types of medical dysfunction. The following is the list of just some of the co-existing conditions reported by the members of the Periodic Paralysis Support Group (550 members at the time of publishing):

cyclic vomiting syndrome - high cholesterol - diabetes type 2 - peripheral polyneuropathy - arachnoids cysts in the brain - loss of peripheral vision - poly cystic ovarian disease – migraines - osteoporosis (bone crush stage in spine and hips) - spina bifida oculta - small brain ischemia - intolerance to most medications - paradoxical effect to most medications – hypoglycemia - intolerance to anesthesia – cataracts – costochondritis - gluten intolerance - fibrocystic disease - esophageal reflux - esophageal hernia – diverticulitis - hearing loss - lactic acidosis - metabolic acidosis – hypoxemia (low

blood oxygen) - restless leg syndrome - stress fracture of the foot - neuroma (nerve tumor) in both feet - painful and tight calf muscles - fibroid tumor (uterus) - ovarian cysts - chronic bladder infections - extremely dry skin – GERD - weak eye muscles – fasciculations - temporomandibular disorders – reflex sympathetic dystrophy - cervical and uterine cancer - uterine and ovarian cysts – vertigo - blood clots – asthma - low set ears - hyper mobile joints – gastritis – syncope - muscle spasms – depression - obsessive compulsive disorder - memory loss (short term) - chronic fatigue – edema - unnamed lumps in breasts - herpes simplex A (lips-cold sores) - gastro paresis – myalgia – myositis – osteoarthritis - myoclonic jerks - dysphagia (trouble swallowing) - lumbar spinal stenosis - many cysts - fatty tumors – hyperthyroid - clotting disorder - memory deficit - compressed pituitary - kidney cyst – allergies – goiter - hardening of the arteries in legs - trouble climbing stairs - low platelet count - mastectomy and hysterectomy - straight spine – vertigo – tinnitus - atrial septal defect - complete heart block – scoliosis pitting edema - thyroid hormone resistance disease - seizures - cluster headaches - severe sleep apnea – rectocele - pulmonary hypertension – candida - acute pancreatitis - chronic pancreatitis - poorly distended bladder - Barrett's esophagus – heart attack - gall bladder issues - carpal tunnel - exercise intolerance - kidney stones - degenerative disk disease - Ehlers-Danlos Syndrome – fibromyalgia - interstitial cystitis - Sjogren's Syndrome – LUPUS - Charcot-Marie Tooth.

Some of these conditions are related to other mutations on chromosome 17, the same chromosome responsible for several forms of Periodic Paralysis. Individuals with genetic mutations on chromosome 17 may also be susceptible to other conditions on the same chromosome. These are often called 'sister' conditions or diseases. An individual with Hypokalemic Periodic Paralysis found at SCN4A on chromosome 17 may also have one or more of over eighty conditions including the following: Malignant Hyperthermia, Ehlers-Danlos Syndrome (EDS), Familial Atrial Fibrillation, Glycogen Storage Disease, Lamb-Girdle Muscular Dystrophy, Paramyotonia Congenita, Potassium-Aggravated Myotonia and possibly other forms of Periodic Paralysis.

It is also known, through research, that some of the other symptoms, diseases and conditions are likely to be related to the Periodic Paralysis. Many of the above conditions are also ion channelopathies, forms of metabolic disorder. They include: fibromyalgia, malignant hyperthermia, chronic fatigue, long QT syndrome, seizures, congenital hypoglycemia, inherited cardiac arrhythmia, migraines, involuntary movement, epilepsy, some autoimmune diseases and hypertension.

Besides having some or all of the complications listed and possible 'sister' conditions, members report having any combination of allergies, autoimmune and inflammatory diseases, conditions and dysfunction (all autoimmune) and surprisingly some mitochondrial dysfunction. Also revealed was what appeared to be a correlation between the length of time an individual had gone without a diagnosis and proper treatment, the number of complications and co-existing conditions they had. Age, lack of time without a diagnosis, misdiagnoses and wrong medications also played a factor. For many, the older the person, the more other complications and conditions existed.

As would be expected, those reporting had more co-existing diseases and conditions and more overall disability and permanent muscle weakness. The other group of individuals with more co-existing conditions was the children of parents who also had Periodic Paralysis. In many, each generation seemed to experience more severe symptoms than the previous generation.

Research indicates that Periodic Paralysis, a metabolic disorder, could cause damage to the mitochondria in the cells. (This may be due to the atypical shifting of potassium.) The damage to the DNA of the mitochondria, in turn contributes to the development of autoimmune disorders. It is our hope that more research will be done in this area, to better be able to recognize and diagnose Periodic Paralysis even though it may co-exist with other conditions and diseases.

The diagnosis and proper treatment of all the forms of Periodic Paralysis in a timely manner is absolutely imperative in order to avoid the possible complications including mitochondrial damage and autoimmune dysfunction and to slow or stop the progression of the disease, which can be permanent.

Unfortunately, the Periodic Paralysis 'specialists' and the 'purists' have not recognized these connections and therefore refuse to diagnose individuals who have diseases or conditions co-existing with the symptoms of Periodic Paralysis. It appears the more conditions that develop; the more difficult it is to recognize the Periodic Paralysis.

ATS-like Characteristics of Periodic Paralysis

Andersen-Tawil Syndrome (ATS) is the most rare form of Periodic Paralysis. It accounts for approximately 10% of all periodic paralysis cases. It is characterized by three particular components: periods of paralysis from high, low or normal potassium levels, distinctive craniofacial and skeletal characteristics and long QT interval heartbeat with a predisposition toward life-threatening ventricular arrhythmia. However, affected individuals may express only one or two of the three components and they may be very subtle. Other characteristics and abnormalities are also associated with Andersen-Tawil Syndrome.

Although these characteristics are associated specifically with Andersen-Tawil Syndrome, many individuals who are diagnosed with other forms also have at least one ATS characteristics. This includes members who were genetically diagnosed with the other forms of Periodic Paralysis. The majority of these characteristics were related to the fingers, toes and facial features.

These findings could not be dismissed as a coincidence. There is a strong possibility that many of the ATS characteristics are quite possibly also seen in the other forms of Periodic Paralysis. Is it possible that these features or traits may have been overlooked in the previous research of patients with other types of Periodic Paralysis?

For this reason, these traits or characteristics as possible more in-depth complications and they may be added to the list of symptoms and characteristics for clinically diagnosing all forms of Periodic Paralysis. This may be essential due to the complications some of these features, like scoliosis, dental anomalies, joint laxity, fused toes or fingers, small jaws or issues with executive functioning may pose.

The Normokalemic Dilemma

The commonly accepted range for normal potassium in human beings is 3.5 to 5.0 mEq/l (milliequivalents per liter), but these numbers may vary somewhat among labs. The human body works to naturally maintain a fine balance, which is within that normal range. Ninety-eight percent of potassium in the body is located within the cells and the other two percent of potassium is outside of the cells in the blood. Blood testing in a lab is used to measure the potassium in the body. There are also a few different types of potassium readers available for purchase and use in the home.

For individuals with Periodic Paralysis, the 'normal' ranges of potassium may vary significantly from person to person. Results from the survey revealed some feel well and are at their best at about 5.0 while others may do best at 3.8 or 4.3. The potassium, for these individuals, shifts in several ways depending on the type of Periodic Paralysis, causing many symptoms as discussed elsewhere in this book. It may shift higher or lower. These shifts may be very slight yet cause paralysis as well as other serious symptoms including but not limited to heart, breathing and blood pressure issues. The shifting may also happen very quickly and be undetectable. This shifting is then within the 'normal' ranges of potassium, thus the name 'Normokalemic' Periodic Paralysis, although some research indicates it is not necessarily a distinct or different form of Periodic Paralysis, but rather Hyperkalemic Periodic Paralysis. However, it appears that about one half of those with all forms of Periodic Paralysis actually have episodes of potassium shifting within normal ranges.

Because most of the emphasis, literature and studies written about Periodic Paralysis are about Hypokalemic Periodic Paralysis (low potassium) and Hyperkalemic Periodic Paralysis (high potassium), the majority of medical professionals do not understand or recognize Normokalemic Periodic Paralysis or the knowledge that the potassium does not have to shift outside of normal ranges or that it may shift too quickly to be detected to create the paralysis or other symptoms which may be serious or life-threatening. It may also shift high or low and return to normal ranges before an individual can be tested in a lab or be seen in the ER.

This makes it difficult when an individual is seeking a diagnosis. Neurologists suspect neurological issues and prescribe very harmful medications, which may cause new symptoms or physical therapy, which can be painful and cause episodes of paralysis. Unfortunately, this may then lead to misdiagnoses of pseudo-seizures, conversion disorder, malingering, attention seeking, and/or hypochondria. More inappropriate and harmful medications and treatments are prescribed to treat these issues. The mis-labels follow the patient from doctor to doctor and the individual is never taken seriously.

These same issues are rampant in an ER situation. Potassium in normal ranges, with paralysis and other issues and uninformed medical professionals, can add up to all of the above and the administration of IV's which are filled with sodium or glucose with a psychotropic drug to treat pseudo seizures. This can lead to more serious symptoms, permanent damage and even death for an individual with Periodic Paralysis.

Another problem resulting from potassium shifting within normal ranges for someone who has a diagnosis of Periodic Paralysis, especially Hypokalemic Periodic Paralysis (low potassium), is the issues of automatically taking a dose of potassium when symptoms begin or being given an IV with potassium in the ER when the potassium never left normal range.

This may then cause a shift into high potassium levels and create new or worse symptoms.

Conversion Disorder vs. Periodic Paralysis

The term 'conversion disorder' (a mental illness) comes up often in conversation among individuals who have Periodic Paralysis. Many have been victims of this mislabel. Due to the potential harm and detriment that this unfortunate diagnosis may bring to the individual with Periodic Paralysis, it is included in this chapter about complications. With each wrong diagnosis, serious and life-threatening complications may arise. Wrong medications due to this unforgivable and unfortunate mistake may be prescribed. Due to a lack of proper treatment, patients get sicker, more damage is done to the organs, permanent muscle weakness sets in and death may occur. This is called iatrogenesis; illness caused directly from a doctor's treatment or lack of appropriate treatment.

As discussed earlier, statistics indicate it takes approximately twenty years for someone to get a diagnosis for Periodic Paralysis. This is inexcusable and is due to several factors as discussed. First, everything else must be ruled out and secondly, because it looks 'fake' to doctors. Nearly every patient with Periodic Paralysis is or has been mislabeled with 'conversion disorder' before they received their diagnosis.

This is just the tip of the iceberg for individuals with Periodic Paralysis. They have unexplained bouts with partial to total body paralysis, which include frightening heart arrhythmia, choking, fluctuating blood pressure and heart rate. While in this state they are unable to communicate, they are given IV's with medications/drugs/compounds, which make it worse.

They are able to hear everything going on as the doctors insist they are faking it, insisting they are having pseudo seizures, pinching them or sticking them with needles to make them respond, demeaning and insulting them and their family members. Conversion disorder is written in the charts and comments like, "refused to lift leg when asked" is written rather than the truth, which is "cannot lift his leg when asked." Some people actually die during these horrific ER or hospital stays and the death certificate may contain any number of false causes.

Conclusion

Most material written about Periodic Paralysis is very simple, basic and limited. That is, that there are several forms and the symptoms; usually episodes of paralysis or muscles weakness, occur due to the improper shifting of potassium. Taking potassium can stop episodes or prevent them and most people live a normal life span without complications. This chapter demonstrates that Periodic Paralysis is much more complex and multifaceted than previously written about in most articles and publications and shared by most researchers and doctors. Many of these complications, issues, symptoms and characteristics are very serious, overlooked and rarely discussed. They need to be recognized and used as part of the diagnostic and treatment process.

This chapter is the most complex for these reasons. Anyone associated with an individual who has a form of Periodic Paralysis must understand that it is more than just periods of paralysis. Any number of other symptoms and complications can and probably will occur, affecting the quality of life of the individual.

Most of it is beyond the individual's control. Understanding these issues is very necessary.

My complex complications:
(You may add your personal information to share with others for their better understanding before you pass along this book.)

Eight

Prognosis For Periodic Paralysis

Expectations For Individuals With Periodic Paralysis

The Effects Of Periodic Paralysis Cannot Be Minimized For Most Of Us

When someone realizes that they have a form of Periodic Paralysis, he or she wants to know what is going to happen. (This is also true for the person's family and friends.) What will the future hold for him or her? Each individual wants to know what to expect. The individual will ask and want the answers to the following questions. How long will I live? How bad will I get? Can this disease be reversed if I get proper treatment? Will I lose my ability to walk? Will I ever drive again? Will I need to be in an assisted living program? Is there medication to stop the total paralytic episodes? What are my chances of dying from the long QT interval heart beat? Will my breathing continue to get more difficult until I can no longer breathe on my own? Is there any medication I can take if I get another bladder infection? What happens if I need an operation and cannot use anesthetics? What can I do to stop the pain in my shoulders and back since I cannot take any pain medications? When I go into cardiac arrest, is it worth trying to save me? Will I end up on dialysis due to kidney failure? Can I travel? What will happen if I end up in the Emergency Room again and they cannot help me with any medications?

The answer is that the affects of Periodic Paralysis cannot be 'minimized' for most of us, both physically and, psychologically. Periodic Paralysis touches every part of our lives, however, it may be different for each individual. There are no absolutes.

For many people with Periodic Paralysis their life span will be normal with very mild symptoms, but for others there may be severe complications and their life may be shortened. For some individuals with Periodic Paralysis, a questionable drug may control the symptoms. For others, however, they are not without side effects. For many more individuals the drugs do not work and are harmful. For most people with Periodic Paralysis the weakness and paralysis are intermittent. There is a beginning and end and between the episodes the individual is normal. Some of these individuals can lead a fairly normal life. However, for many individuals the quality of life is compromised and the weakness can linger or become permanent. Some of them will become disabled and debilitated, require the use of a power wheelchair and will probably be unable to work a job or have a career. They will spend much of their time in bed or in a recliner, unable to do much more. They will need assistance with and for all parts of their lives. In some rare cases, Periodic Paralysis can cause a sudden, untimely or early death.

For many who have this condition, when they are not in paralysis, they are in a state of disabling fatigue and overwhelming weakness or abortive attacks much of the time. Their minds experience a brain fog, and the potassium shifting can cause depression or anxiety, changes in personality, and many other long time issues like kidney stones and osteoporosis. The medications prescribed for Periodic Paralysis for many of them, either do not work or make symptoms worse. They cannot take other medications to treat the side effects or the possible accompanying conditions. They try everything and anything to stop this. They research and study looking for answers. They join support groups seeking support, understanding and validation. They share their stories and experiences hoping others who are going through the same things may have information about a new drug or a new idea or a new treatment.

Every once in awhile, an individual will have a great day and almost feel normal. At those times he or she pushes himself or herself and plays catch-up for chores, work, school, family or hobbies and then returns to the debilitating symptoms once again, because they did push themself. Most of the time they do not know what made them have a good day or what made them worse again. Others, like family members, neighbors, friends, and teachers, may not understand and mistake this for 'faking,' 'making it up' or being 'lazy.' Periodic Paralysis is cruel and unpredictable. The people around those with Periodic Paralysis need to understand this and believe that their loved one is doing the best he or she can.

This also applies to the doctors working with these individuals. This is devastating and adds to the cruelty of the disease. The reality and truth is, due to the lack of understanding and recognition of Periodic Paralysis by medical professionals, many of the people with this medical condition will end up very, very ill due to the lack of a diagnosis. They are misdiagnosed, under diagnosed, called hypochondriacs, or mentally ill. They are diagnosed as suffering from conversion disorder, or having pseudo seizures. They are laughed at and scoffed at. They are told they are "too old" or it is not possible because they are "black." They are told Periodic Paralysis is "too rare" for them to have it. They are mistreated with medications that make them worse. Doctors dismiss them and ridicule them and lie about them in the medical records. They do not get the medication or treatments they need. Then they die of things such as, 'unknown' muscle wasting disease, accidental drowning in a pool or bathtub, cardiac arrest at age 40, stroke, or failure to thrive. The worst is from suicide. Some may just give up, because if the doctors do not believe that one is really ill, how can family members be expected to believe it?

It is essential that more doctors become aware of Periodic Paralysis and that they be taught more about the condition in medical school. The information should be correct and up-to-date. They should understand that anyone might have a rare medical condition. Medical professionals need to learn to recognize, diagnose and treat it in a timely manner. Doctors must learn to treat individuals with Periodic Paralysis with respect. Until then, however, the patients with this condition will have to take the lead on their own care.

The Best One Can Be

The good news is, that although there is no certainty that someone can obtain a diagnosis and that there is no simple pill or magical cure for Periodic Paralysis, there is HOPE for a better life! As explained earlier in this book, for most individuals the paralysis and some of the symptoms can be controlled and managed by following a plan of common sense and natural methods, even without a diagnosis. If an individual realizes that he or she has a form of Periodic Paralysis and seeks help before a diagnosis is established (and after of course), one can experience some relief by making some lifestyle changes.

This is not to say, however, that each person can or will be cured or never have another symptom or episode of weakness or paralysis. It simply means they may be able to reduce the number of paralytic episodes or muscle weakness, the length of the attacks and the intensity of them and reduce some of the symptoms. The episodes will still occur, just not as severely and not as often. Each individual will still have muscle damage, permanent muscle weakness, exercise intolerance, abortive attacks, the inability to work or more, depending upon one's already present condition, age, coexisting conditions and amount of damage already done. They will, however, feel better in some ways and have a better quality of life.

Each individual with Periodic Paralysis has the opportunity to be the best he or she can be and improve the quality of his or her life by individualizing their own plan based on what works for them and the ideas in this book (and the other PPN books as well as in the PPN Forum). The sooner an individual begins to follow the appropriate plan for his or her individual needs and condition, the sooner they can and will do better and may live a longer and healthier life.

There is HOPE for those with Periodic Paralysis.

Nine

Conclusion

Conclusion

Awareness

Due to the reasons addressed throughout this book in the previous chapters, there needs to be more awareness of Periodic Paralysis. When the terms multiple sclerosis, muscular dystrophy, ALS (Lou Gehrig's disease), cancer or leukemia are heard someone automatically visualizes an individual whose health is compromised, probably in some pain, maybe in a wheelchair and unable to go about normal daily duties unaided. The futures of these individuals are uncertain. Most people are moved to sadness and concern for those individuals. Family, friends, churches, and even entire neighborhoods and communities readily offer help and support.

When someone suffering the effects of the cruel condition of Periodic Paralysis mentions the term 'Periodic Paralysis' blank stares and lack of understanding are the norm. Very few people on earth have heard of it or know about it. This needs to be changed.

When the words 'Periodic Paralysis' are heard everyone should instantly visualize an individual becoming suddenly totally paralyzed, unable to walk or talk and in fear because his or her heart is racing and beating irregularly, blood pressure is dangerously high or low, breathing is difficult and may stop, oxygen may be very low, choking may occur, and he or she may die during the episode from a heart arrhythmia and/or respiratory or cardiac arrest. He or she looks asleep or unconscious, but can hear everything going on, but cannot say a word. The individual is vulnerable and at the mercy of others and 'totally alone in the dark.' Over time, gradual, permanent muscle weakness sets in and the person becomes disabled. The future of these individuals is as uncertain as in the other conditions.

Hopefully, this can and will be changed with the information shared and contained in this book. It is time to come out of the dark ages as far as Periodic Paralysis is concerned. The world needs to know about the forms of Periodic Paralysis. Many people have it without realizing it. They are misdiagnosed and suffering greatly from the mistreatment they are now receiving. The more awareness there is, the better chance of it being recognized and diagnosed properly.

It is our greatest hope and desire that this booklet, *What Is Periodic Paralysis? A Disease Like No Other,* can be a tool or an instrument that will bring awareness to the rare and disabling mineral metabolic disorder known as Periodic Paralysis. We hope that those who read it will be educated in and better understand all aspects of Periodic Paralysis, including but not limited to the symptoms, the diagnosis and the treatment.

Conclusion

This chapter and book will conclude by sharing the thoughts and words of individuals, who live with, struggle with and suffer from Periodic Paralysis each and every day; the members of our 'Periodic Paralysis Network Support, Education and Advocacy Group.' They responded to the following the question:

"What is the most important thing you want the world to know about Periodic Paralysis?"

The following are their heartfelt answers:

Periodic Paralysis exists.
~

There is not a cure yet!
~

Periodic Paralysis is a real disability.
~

It affects the entire family.
~

I don't have conversion disorder!!! That this is a real horrifying, terrifying and totally unpredictable disease that I wouldn't wish on my worst enemy! That I feel like I'm drowning in a pool with one hand sticking out crying..."HELP ME!"
~

Periodic Paralysis is life altering, devastating, and cruel.
~

I want them to know I won't get better; it is always there with me. In every activity I do. Periodic Paralysis is there in my body telling me, "Here I am." "Go slower" or "Stop." Even on a day that I look good and am smiling, Periodic Paralysis is there ready to come out. Every task makes me tired and is an effort. But, we do live, smile, laugh, go and come, even though there is a sickness within us. But, I am not better; there is no cure. I am just alive like you.

~

I want them to know that there are times the 'PP' people look, act and feel fine but it can drastically change in the blink of an eye - literally. Two examples:

My husband, who has Hypokalemic Periodic Paralysis, was going to put the spare tire back on the rack under the bed of my truck. It requires lying just a bit under the truck to guide the wrench onto the pulley/riser slot to the right place then crank. He was strong, feeling fine when he laid down, fine when he reached up to guide the wrench into the slot but by the time I'd made one turn of the wrench, he was in full body paralysis. I, as caregiver, had to drag him out enough to sit him up and give him emergency potassium. I had to hold him up in place until he was able to breath well, move and roll over

We were sitting at the computer playing solitaire. He clicked the showing Ace and commented, "Get up there." Before he could roll the arrow down about 8 inches, he dropped into full body paralysis requiring, again, emergency potassium drink.

Conclusion

We won't talk about those episodes when he was carrying something...

~

I would like people to know its not my fault and that I can't make it better by getting in shape.

~

It is a lonely illness!

~

I panic when someone asks me to make plans and hate having to use my disability as an excuse. I've avoided having to organize anything for years. I always wonder if people think I am lazy but just the thought of organizing things makes me exhausted.

~

It's more than 'just' paralysis. It's pain, weakness, physical and mental exhaustion that others can't understand.

~

I want them to know that "Eat more bananas" doesn't work...

~

I want them to know that the caregivers for someone with PP can't just suddenly 'go shopping' or 'spend an afternoon at the park' or 'go see a movie with me' or 'make plans for next weekend'. We also have to cancel plans we had because our PP rebel isn't feeling strong. We need people to understand we're not making excuses. Yes we may end up sitting and watching TV all evening or we could be required to dose emergency meds, handle or move a person in attack to a safe or comfortable spot while monitoring vitals, dress a wound caused from a sudden attack; even be required to perform rescue breathing or CPR.

∼

It is a real disease- it isn't in our heads. Although I might look ok I'm usually just trying to keep on going for the sake of my family and my girls.

∼

I want people to know there are good days and bad days. Just because I worked circles around everyone yesterday doesn't mean I'll be able to today. Over excursion can burn up the next day due to continuing to push harder and harder.

∼

I want the medical field to be required to know about Periodic Paralysis. Often times in the ER no one even knows what it is, which in turn can be life threatening for us

∼

Potassium does not have to shift out of normal levels in all forms of PP or go below normal (especially very low) in Hypokalemic Periodic Paralysis to cause symptoms or severe paralysis that can last for hours.

∼

I was misdiagnosed for 30 years and just 3 years ago got the proper diagnosis but still have to experience ignorance in the medical field. I actually had one neurologist tell me he didn't study on PP because he knew it was impossible he would encounter it in his career. Obviously it's not as rare as they believe. It's just misdiagnosed for many, many years.

Conclusion

For so long we don't have any idea what's going on with our bodies, then we get some relief when we find out it has a name "Periodic Paralysis" or "PP" for short, but then we start educating ourselves. We learn, there is no cure, and how complicated it is. We feel alone, we have to start asking for help, and no one understands, even the doctors. We grieve our old lives and that includes our dreams, hobbies, and independence. Most of all it affects our family too. Worst of all most of us will end up needing a caregiver.

∼

To our loved ones and friends...please stay with us...it is not something that goes away quickly...it is lonely...we need you long term....

∼

It makes you feel worthless because a lot of people don't understand. They tell you just have to push yourself and don't really believe you. You make plans with someone and then can't go and you feel guilty. It is very lonely.

∼

We need better treatment in the ER.

∼

It feels like you are not control of your body and an alien took over.

∼

I want my family to believe in Periodic Paralysis and to believe that I have it. I want them to know that some of them may have it too. They also may be carriers.

∼

It's devastating, cruel and affects the whole family. It is there, waiting in the background to make a strike to ruin my day. Eating bananas or getting in shape won't help. Just because I don't look sick doesn't mean I am not. It can't be controlled and I don't have a crystal ball to predict my episodes. I need understanding from people when I have to cancel plans because I am having an episode or too tired after a severe one. Please understand I didn't choose it, I was born with it.

~

Even though you are unable to respond to people, you can still feel and hear and you are still a human being. Please remember that.

~

I don't like to make plans. I never know what tomorrow has in store

~

I am a person and my disease does not define me.

~

Honestly, it has to be one of the most cruel and misunderstood diseases. It can hit someone out of the blue, trap you in an aborted episode, destroy fitness, relationships, make it impossible to do what was once easy, and makes you a target for ignorant doctors, particularly the arrogant ones who must always be right- and their attitude can literally kill you. I don't normally say much, but this question brought back every bad and terrifying experience that has gone with it.

~

Conclusion

People with Periodic Paralysis can and do have pain.

~

I want the world to know that our bodies will do things doctors weren't taught in medical school. Doing tests, not finding an answer does not equal a psychological diagnosis. Depression and anxiety are real. Just because lots of friends and family have depression doesn't mean I have it because my labs and tests came back normal. Out of 26 labs, most in the hospital and the ER, only 6 times ever was my potassium checked, 4 were low enough for hypokalemia. Only once was I given potassium after being checked. My doctors thought all that time all electrolytes were being checked. They were told "normal electrolytes" results by hospital doctors when only magnesium was checked. It was misleading. This prevented me from getting correct treatment of more potassium.

~

Periodic Paralysis is a mineral metabolic disorder not a neurological disorder.

~

I always felt it important to be dependable. It stresses and frustrates me that it's hard to commit to things, knowing that one second or one variable can totally change the day and I must cancel and take time to recover.

~

Food can be effectively used as medicine and it feels so much better than severe reactions to most prescriptions.

~

At the very least the clinicians and providers at MDA clinics should be well versed with ACCURATE information since this organization and their clinics are considered the 'go-to' for diagnosis since PP is one of conditions 'under their umbrella' and research money is given to them.

It is also reasonable to be able to expect and depend on MDA to live up to their statements about providing services and support to individuals and families to have more in depth and breadth of accurate information about PP. And be humble enough to realize and admit that there is still a lot of 'missing'/'unknown' information about PP. Let alone that no one person, even with knowing so much and more than many other providers, can know what is known about PP and can have enough knowledge because it's so complex.

~

Most of us are afraid of the ER. We fear being treated with an IV or an anesthesia that could harm us.

~

When dealing with patients with Periodic Paralysis, it seems like too many in the medical field don't implement applying 'Patient Rights' in their attitude, tone and temperament. It states that as patients we have the right to be treated with dignity and respect (not defensive, hostile, disdainful, derogatory, demeaning doctors and others)... And worse, we get so intimidated and threatened (especially when not well) and afraid of retaliation (what they might say/write in notes about us) that we don't confront them and in essence 'allow' them to act as if they can treat and talk to us in whatever way they want and we have to accept it.

~

You have made my day. For years I had no validation of this body. This question and all the answers you all give is the best thing to happen in years. Every response I read was me. Like you are looking into my soul and letting me know this is all real. It is so empowering!!!!! What a great question.
Wish we could have a convention and meet you all but in reality none of us could come. Thank you all, you bring order to my chaos!!!!!

~

Thank you to the members of our PPN Support Group. We remain ever hopeful! This book is for you!!!

For more information about Periodic Paralysis:
The following are the services and features of our PPN forum:

PPN Website: **www.periodicparalysisnetwork.com**

PPN Books:
Living With Periodic Paralysis: The Mystery Unraveled
https://www.createspace.com/4111713

The Periodic Paralysis Guide And Workbook: Be The Best You Can Be Naturally
https://www.createspace.com/4326356

A Bill Of Rights For Periodic Paralysis Patients
https://www.createspace.com/5705192

(Also found on our website)
http://www.periodicparalysisnetwork.com/books.htm

PPN Blog: **http://livingwithperiodicparalysis.blogspot.com/**

PPN Support, Education and Advocacy Group:
https://www.facebook.com/groups/periodicparalysisnetworksupportgroup/

PPN Book Discussion Group:
https://www.facebook.com/groups/periodicparalysisnetwork/

PPN Genealogy Discussion Group:
https://www.facebook.com/groups/580168915344191/

PPNI Genetics Discussion and Research Group.
https://www.facebook.com/groups/1574048096186578/

Periodic Paralysis Caregivers:
https://www.facebook.com/groups/366386850151623/

The PPN Learning Center and Workshop:
https://www.facebook.com/groups/1416848568618404/

PPN Website Facebook Page:
https://www.facebook.com/PeriodicParalysisNetwork

PPN Author's Page:
https://www.facebook.com/SusanQKnittleHunterauthor

Email: **periodicparalysisnetwork@gmail.com**

Fund raisers:
GoFundMe: **http://www.gofundme.com/ftnr50**
Bravelets: **https://www.bravelets.com/bravepage/alone-in-the-dark-periodic-paralysis**

PPN Members World Map:
http://www.multiplottr.com/?map_id=55083

About the Author and Co-Founders of the Periodic Paralysis Network, Inc.

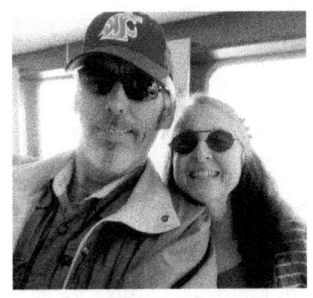

Calvin and Susan Q. Knittle-Hunter are the co-creators, co-founders and co-directors of the Periodic Paralysis Network, Inc. (PPNI), which is an independent, educational corporation, designed to provide support, education and advocacy to individuals with Periodic Paralysis.

Susan, the Managing Director of PPNI, earned B.S. degrees in Psychology and Special Education at the University of Utah and spent many years as a teacher and case manager working with children and adults with disabilities. She suffers from the rare and disabling mineral metabolic disorder called Periodic Paralysis.

Calvin, the Primary Director of PPNI, earned B.S. degrees in Behavioral Science and Psychology at Westminster College and the University of Utah. He also holds a M.Ed. degree in Special Education and M.S. degree in Information Technology from the University of Utah and Capella University. Calvin worked in a variety of fields including teaching, corrections and case management.

Calvin and Susan have co-authored and co-published five books; *Living With Periodic Paralysis: The Mystery Unraveled*, *The Periodic Paralysis Guide and Workbook: Be The Best You Can Be Naturally*, *A Bill Of Rights For Periodic Paralysis Patients*, *Sotos Syndrome: A Tribute to Sandy* and *Moments In Time: At Home In The Woods*.

The tree reflects the single "Tree of Life" those of us with Periodic Paralysis share. The earth signifies the elements: potassium, magnesium, sodium, etc. The broken earth signifies the break in those for us. Created by Calvin Hunter.
Periodic Paralysis Network, Inc
Copyright © 2016

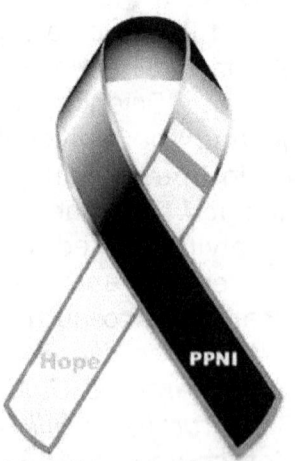

The Awareness Ribbon for Periodic Paralysis is cream and silver. Cream is the color of the Awareness Ribbon for paralysis and silver is the color of potassium. Created by Susan Q. Knittle-Hunter.
Periodic Paralysis Network, Inc
Copyright © 2016

Notes

Notes

www.ingramcontent.com/pod-product-compliance
Lightning Source LLC
Chambersburg PA
CBHW070322190526
45169CB00005B/1700